365 HEALTH AND FITNESS HACKS THAT COULD SAVE YOUR LIFE

JOEY THURMAN, CPT, FNS, BLS

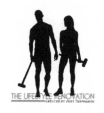

THE LIFESTYLE RENOVATION

The information provided in this book is for educational purposes only. Joey Thurman is not a doctor and information in this book is not meant to be taken as medical advice. The information provided is based upon Joey's experiences as well as his interpretations of the current research available.

The advice and tips given are meant for healthy adults only. You should consult your physician to ensure tips given in this book are appropriate for your individual circumstances.

If you have any health issues or pre-existing conditions, please consult with your Physician before implementing any of the information provided.

This product is for informational purposes only and the author does not accept any responsibilities for any liabilities or damages, real or perceived, resulting from the use of this information.

365 Health and Fitness Hacks That Could Save Your Life

Copyright ©2016 Frederic Joseph Thurman

All copyrights are reserved.

Printed and distributed by Bookbaby™

ISBN: 978-1-48356-101-1 (Print)
ISBN: 978-1-48356-102-8 (eBook)

Acknowledgments

I want to thank all of my current and former clients for the privilege of knowing you and allowing me to beat you up in the gym. I want to thank my family and friends for always believing in me and being by my side. Thanks Mom and Dad for always believing in your "little" boy! Thanks to Terrence Howard, Chef Art Smith, Dr. Laura Berman, and Dr. Paul Savage for their amazing quotes! Thanks to Frank Martinelli for the book cover design (Imfmproductions.com), Erik Johnson for shooting the cover (Residualscars.com), and Greg Vaughan for my bio picture (Gregvaughanstudio.com). Thanks to my father-in-law for his advice throughout this process.

Thanks to my brother from another mother Marcus Warren. Your constant encouragement and belief has led me to become a better fitness expert and man.

Most of all, a big thank you to my amazing wife Maria! You are my heart, my soul, my life! Thank you for always being by my side through the ups and more importantly downs! You are my strength when I am weak!
Love you always and forever!

TABLE OF CONTENTS

INTRODUCTION

We want, we want, we want but when our wants actually require putting forth hard work, we resort to complaining about what we can't have. Then when someone offers a solution to our problems, rather than accepting it, we make up excuses. For example, we claim it's too hard or say that we'll try (starting on Monday of course), but we never take action. In reality, we aren't willing to make the changes in our lives that we are complaining about, we choose not to better ourselves, and we would rather sit and complain about what 'could be' rather than going out there and achieving it. What if we stopped complaining and changed the way we looked at our lives, our health, and our bodies?

Imagine that you have an old house, you have owned this house for years and it's full of memories, good and bad. You LOVE this house but you are getting tired of seeing the same dull paint, the same layout, or hearing the same squeaky door that you have been meaning to fix for several years! You don't want to give up on the house...so don't! It's imperative to provide your house with continuous TLC so it doesn't crumble to the ground before its time. You need to REMODEL and RENOVATE it from the inside out! But instead of immediately taking a sledgehammer to every wall in the house without rhyme or reason, it's important to develop a plan. Ask yourself; where will my motivation come from? What are the issues and what are my goals? What steps do I need to take? What will the final product look like? Sure you can make a house look nice from the outside, with new landscaping and home décor, because appearance makes an impression, but if you don't address the issues that lie underneath the fresh coat of paint, you are setting your house, and yourself, up for failure. You must assess your base, the foundation, to make your house as strong as possible. You will then need to focus on the framework and ask yourself what internal improvements are going to make your house run as efficiently as possible. Maybe it's a new kitchen, windows, roof or a new layout. Now, think of this house as you, your body, your health, your life!

We all want a quick fix to all of our problems, and getting healthy is no exception. If there was only a magical pill to fix our every ill; but until then we will have to put in good old fashioned hard work! Hard work is imperative for overall success, but most of us spread ourselves pretty thin and the thought of making a change may seem overwhelming; especially if we are unsure as to where to begin. So that's where I come in; to provide you with more efficient ways to get your health back on track that you can realistically incorporate in your everyday life. We need to get away from being OVERFED and UNDERNOURISHED and use the tools in this book to provide our body with the continuous TLC it so desperately needs.

You can use this book however you wish; you don't necessarily have to read through the entire book front to back in one sitting. Take a look at the contents and find the best sections that apply to you and your scenario. This book will give you tips and tricks….or 'HACKS' to make yourself healthier, happier, more efficient, and ultimately save your life! Why not keep this book at your bedside table and read a few tips every day? Use it as a hub of useful information; or a Do-It-Yourself go to guide, that you can refer back to at any point. Some hacks may provide different strategies and methods (like a full body workout vs. split body workout) so it's about finding what hacks work best for you and your life. Let today be the first step to a brighter and healthier future and let this book be your 'bible of knowledge' to keep as a reference. Enjoy the journey!

THE DEMOLITION: CLEARING EXERCISE

1) CLEAR YOUR MIND!

So you have decided to make a change towards a heathier, brighter future; GREAT! But where do you start? I always suggest, before anything else, to take part in a clearing exercise. When you make a big change to your life, your mindset is one of the most important things to consider. The second you start to doubt yourself, you have lost. You need to remove all negative thoughts and replace them with positive ones!

The first step towards this is to make a list of all the negatives in your life. This can be ABSOLUTELY ANYTHING; it could be something that you don't like about yourself (e.g. your love handles), those feelings and thoughts that you wouldn't dare to tell anyone, or worries about your future. Any worries you have or negative thoughts that you encounter, write them down; no one is judging you for this and neither should you!

Next, create a second list made up entirely of positive thoughts. Write down your positive attributes, dreams and aspirations! I know you have them because you are reading this book right now! It may be weight that you want to lose or to simply look better in your birthday suit. You may want to gain more confidence to impress the new object of your desires. It may be career based or something to do with your family. Whatever it is, no matter how crazy, if it's positive, WRITE IT DOWN. You now have the two lists sitting in front of you and it is time to choose your new path to positivity.

This next step is fun and incredibly satisfying; it is time to get rid of those negative thoughts. Pick up the piece of paper with your negative thoughts and rip it, shred it, or maybe even BURN it! I don't care how you do it, just GET RID OF IT! Remove it from your life; remove all the negativity that has been weighing you down.

Didn't that feel good!? How easy it was to get rid of all of those negative thoughts and feelings. Now that they are gone you are in control of your life. It is time to focus on the future and the person that you WANT to be. Keep the positive list and look at it regularly. Whenever you feel bad and find yourself in a funk take out your positive sheet of goals; look at it and remember why you have decided to make a better life for yourself. Make sure you keep sight of your goals at all times because it is easy to lose them in this busy world in which we live. We are only on this planet once so live out your dreams!

THE DESIGN: GOAL SETTING AND MOTIVATION

2) READY, SET, GOAL!

'I don't need to set goals' or 'Targets are pointless' are just two statements that I have heard recently which are complete and utter RUBBISH. The avoidance of goal setting makes us prone to accepting less than what we want, it allows us to SETTLE, but we don't want to settle, we want to GROW AND SUCCEED. Only THREE out of every 100 people actually write down their goals on a piece of paper. I cannot express how vital it is to have goals, and more importantly, to write them down and devise a plan of how to work towards them. If you do not set goals for yourself, you do not have an aim, and therefore have no motivation to keep on a diet or to keep exercising. So why not grab a piece of paper and write down 3 things that you want to achieve from this book in the next month. For example; you may want to lose 7 pounds before that wedding in a few weeks or you may want to train enough to be able to run 5 miles next month. Your goal can be anything and it is COMPLETELY UNIQUE to you! It could even be something as simple as making use of your free time more efficiently. For example, you could start by exercising instead of watching TV for the two hours of spare time you have after work. Goals that are kept and engrained in one's mind are less likely to get mixed up with the other 1,500 thoughts per minute that the average human has…yes 1,500! No wonder so many people lose sight of what they are trying to achieve! Write down your goals right now and stick them on a wall or to your fridge so you are constantly reminded of the person you want to be……and CAN be!

I am now going to share some tips, or hacks, with you that will guide you on this journey, help with your goal setting as well as your motivation! So keep on reading and I am confident that you will be successful in making this change you have decided for yourself!

3) SAY HI TO S.A.M.!

This is one of the most important tips I can give anyone; you must set goals which are Specific, Achievable, and Measurable (S.A.M)! This is so simple yet so important; you have to make certain that you pick goals that are realistic and suited to you. It's great to have goals and dreams. Dreams give us hope, they give us light; but when that light it too far away and unattainable, we set ourselves up for disappointment. It's great to say that you are going to do something, like get healthy; however, nothing is accomplished without first setting a specific and realistic goal. Sure, I would love to wake up in the morning and be able to run a marathon and finish without breaking a sweat; but life doesn't work that way. We aren't children anymore and, for example, we cannot dream to be astronauts and simultaneously professional hockey players as I did when I was a child. We must develop short and long-range plans that are appropriately comprehensive, realistic, and effective in meeting our goals.

As a health and fitness expert, I regularly hear people say 'I gave up' or 'I just couldn't do it, it was impossible.' I then ask them what their aim was, what it was that they wanted to achieve. They reply, 'I wanted to run 10 miles at once by the end of the week', yet they haven't gone for a run since they were in gym class 20 years ago. THIS IS NOT REALISTIC! Let's say your goal is to run 10 miles without stopping. That's great, but you must first develop a plan and choose a suitable and realistic time frame in order to achieve this goal; let's say two or three months. Then, you can split the main goal into little challenges. Identify a few intermediate but critical success factors that you can realistically accomplish towards achieving your overall goal. For example, it may be wise to set daily, weekly, and monthly goals as follows:

- ✓ Day 1 – finish 1 mile even if you have to walk part of the time

- ✓ End of week 1- run 1 mile without stopping

- ✓ End of month 1 – run 3 miles without stopping

- ✓ End of month 2 – run 7 miles without stopping

- ✓ End of month 3 – run 10 miles without stopping

Now it's great that you managed to run ten miles, but you want to get yourself into a position where you can run ten miles CONSISTENTLY, time and time again, not just once!

4) ON THE RIGHT TRACK!

Keep a compelling scoreboard. People play differently when they are keeping score. This can be vital in helping to motivate you on a daily/weekly basis. It may be wise to invest in a dry-erase board or journal (if you prefer to write things down) or use your smartphone (if you are more tech savvy) where you can chart how well you are doing. If you aim is to lose 14 pounds before a certain date, you can use the board to set specific targets and then compare your actual progress as you go. For example, you may want to lose one or two pounds a week. Monitor your progress each week by logging your actual weight next to your target. If you have achieved your short term goal that's great; you will feel better for it. You will even be more motivated to continue because you can see, and more importantly, **feel** the positive changes in your life! If you are not doing so well against your target, use it as motivation to try harder and/or reassess the steps you are taking to reach your goal. People too often see not hitting a goal as back tracking and they use this as an excuse to give up. Don't let this get you down; use this as your fuel to continue on your journey and SHOW YOURSELF that you CAN DO THIS and try EVEN HARDER next week!

5) TALK IS CHEAP, START NOW!

It is so easy to postpone taking action; how many times have you said 'oh, I'm going to start next week' or 'I'm starting on Monday'. WHY WAIT? START NOW! What is so special about Monday anyway? 'Joey I'm going to start eating healthier in a few weeks, but until then I will eat whatever I want!' Why make things harder on yourself!? The most popular example of this is the start of the New Year; it can be fantastic to set yourself a goal for the year ahead, but in reality 92% of resolutions fail by January 15th. It is great that you changed your life for two weeks, but what if you could change your life forever? I believe that new year's resolutions set us up for failure because they are not well planned and are typically abandoned very quickly; besides you won't feel so bad about giving up since its what's 'supposed' to happen! Realistically, if you are putting off your goal, saying you'll start in two weeks rather than today, it may be because you don't really have the focus or true intention to achieve it. Talk is cheap, and you should give yourself more credit. If you really want to change your life, there is no better time than NOW to take action!

6) USE THE BUDDY SYSTEM!

This isn't always needed but people who have a friend by their side going through the same challenges are more likely to succeed (assuming your friend does not display behaviors that will impact your motivation and set you back). This is because you can encourage, help, support, and keep each other accountable for achieving results. There may be days when you struggle to find the motivation to 'get up and go.' However, a friend who has common goals relying on you to be successful can be the catalyst in providing you with the extra strength and motivation to not give up. If you let yourself down you also let your partner down; and vice versa. Make a competition between the two of you so you can continually motivate one another! If you don't have a partner, do not to worry, we have technology. Get online and find someone who is willing to work out with you; make a posting on Facebook, talk to people at work, or use an app like *Pillar* to help you find fitness partners and coaches for likeminded people. LOVE THIS!

7) FOCUS ON THE POSITIVE!

When completing a major change in your life, the easiest thing to do is to focus on the negatives; let me rephrase that, the LAZIEST thing to do is to focus on the negatives. You need to change your mindset and start to focus on the positives instead! Think about your end goal and why you are doing it in the first place! For example, instead of thinking about the unhealthy foods you will be LOSING, think about all the wonderful foods you will be GAINING. Think about all the new recipes you can try, and how all of the healthy foods that you normally walk passed in the supermarket can transform your meals!

8) REMOVE NEGATIVITY!

I'm not just talking about negative thoughts and feelings; I'm talking about negative PEOPLE! You have chosen to change your life but you have to remember that not all people have the positivity that you do! You don't need those people! All they will do is bring you down and make you feel worthless. Let the people around you know that you are making a healthy lifestyle change and you need their support, not their negativity. If they don't agree with your decision and act in a manner that can derail your progress, they are NOT worth your time or energy! Sure, it would be ideal if your positivity was contagious and inspired them to make a change, but more often than not, unfortunately, this is not the case. Make sure you surround yourself with positive people who want to see you succeed so you keep your motivation levels high and cut those non-achievers loose!

9) NO ONE IS FORCE FEEDING YOU!

A lot of people tend to force themselves to eat foods that they don't like because they are healthy, that's great that you are eating healthy food but if you don't like them this is NEVER going to work! You won't have any motivation to carry on eating foods you hate! The excuse 'I don't really like healthy foods' is no longer valid because there are SO MANY options available. The internet has a mecca of healthy recipes you can try! Make trying new things fun and exciting! This way, your efforts will be more sustainable and you are more likely to stick to your goal! (Healthy recipes included in this book.)

10) BOOTY BANK!

What makes the world go round? MONEY! You can try and motivate yourself by setting up an 'Exercise Jar', 'Booty Bank' (ha…get it?), or whatever label you give it to motivate you. Every time you work out or every day you avoid unhealthy foods (it may be your favorite chocolate cake or bag of chips), put some money in the jar. Since the average person makes 200 decisions about food every day it can add up quickly! If you set a reward for yourself, you will have the incentive to earn it! For example, when I reach $50, I will treat myself to a new pair of shoes. You have to be tough as well as honest with yourself on this one and maybe even include a penalty if you go against your system. If you fail, you are only cheating yourself! Failure is NOT acceptable!

11) FORWARD THINKING!

There's no point in dwelling on the past. What you can do is LEARN from it! So leave the past where it is, live in the present, and prepare for your future. It's wise to utilize this mentality when it comes to your health. Always remember your end goal! Make sure you read the goal(s) you have written down on a daily basis; which can be a great tool to re-energize you to go again! If you do fall down a path of having a bad meal, hour, day, or even week (yes it happens) tell yourself that it's not over, you CAN and WILL achieve your goals!

12) ELIMINATE THE BACK UP PLAN!

YOU have decided this goal for yourself for a reason! There should be no 'backup plan' that allows you not to hit this target. If you say 'well if I don't hit my goal, I will be happy with slightly less', you are already starting with the wrong mindset. BE POSITIVE! Tell yourself that you are going to hit the target and that you are going to work hard at it, AND THAT'S IT! Don't settle for anything less! You may be surprised how far you can get when you set the bar high.

THE RESTORATION: THE IMPORTANCE OF SLEEP

'We can sleep when we are dead' is the saying; right? WRONG! Too many people these days miss out on vital sleeping hours and seem to forget just how important sleep can be. Sleep is just as important as any other part of your life and possibly the MOST important thing you can do for your health! Both the quantity and the quality of sleep play a vital role in your overall health and wellbeing.

Sleep is the only time that your body gets to fully relax and re-energize. There is a reason why you wake up feeling tired when you haven't had enough quality sleep; your body hasn't had enough time to recuperate and get ready for the next day! According to a study carried out at Stanford University, college football players who slept OVER 10 HOURS per night for eight weeks, experienced an improvement in their average sprint time as well as greater stamina and less daytime fatigue [8]. A similar test was also carried out on tennis players and swimmers with the same results.

Furthermore, sleep allows you to achieve a process called 'consolidation'. Your body may be relaxed while you are asleep, but your mind is surprisingly active; and this can help when you are learning something new. For example, if you are learning a new topic at school or you are learning a new language, sleep will help to cement everything you have learned (when awake) into your brain!

Everyone wants to live longer, right? That's why you have decided to read this book, because you wanted to make a positive change to your life. Well, sleep can actually help you live longer! It is thought that people who cut short their sleeping hours may also be shortening their lives. Interestingly, this can also happen to people who sleep too much, crazy right? It's all about balance; 7-9 hours of sleep per day is the perfect amount for the average adult who wants to stay healthy!

Sleep also reduces the risk of some health problems! C-reactive protein is normally associated with heart attack risk and the levels of this tend to be higher in people that get less than SIX HOURS of sleep [7]. Achieving the recommended amount of sleep is also said to decrease inflammation; inflammation can ultimately cause arthritis, diabetes and heart disease. If you thought that sleep wasn't important before, I hope you are starting to now think otherwise!

Finally, a little known fact about the human body is that sleep and metabolism are controlled by the same area of the brain! As a direct result, those that get a healthy amount of sleep find it significantly easier to lose weight. When we are tired our hormones go up in our blood, the same hormones that drive our appetite!

So this all sounds good and I'm sure you have yawned your way through these few sleep paragraphs (and not because you were bored…right?) and are wondering how to fix your sleeping if you struggle to sleep in the first place. Don't worry, I have you covered! Let's take a look at some tips to maximize the benefits of your sleep as well as help you drift off in no time!

Hacks for a Good Night's Sleep

13) HOW LONG SHOULD I SLEEP?

Every single human being in the world is completely different; some people may be able to function on seven hours of sleep whereas others may not be able to function with anything less than eight. Find a pattern that fits you, over the next two weeks, try and be strict with your sleep (even on weekends; waking up early on a Sunday, ugh I know!) and see how you benefit from different amounts of sleep.

14) 90-MINUTE RULE!

Wouldn't it be perfect if we woke up at the perfect time, peacefully, ready for the day ahead! Well, now we can! Research has told us that we sleep in 90 minute brain cycles and that we are closest to our normal waking state at the end of each cycle [10]. There are two ways to do this; first, if you have a time that you want to wake up, count back in 90 minute increments to work out what time you should be going to sleep; this is obviously a rough guide but it should help. The second way is by using your mobile phone or smart watch to track your sleep. There are now several apps that track your sleep and will set off an alarm at the 'right' time to wake you up. Now of course, this is no good if it wakes you up and you're late for work, so you can set a time period (e.g.

between 7:00 and 7:30a.m) and the alarm will go off at the most beneficial moment within that time-frame. Another thing to note is that the app will normally tell you to put the phone under your pillow, which hasn't necessarily been proven to be harmful to your health, but it is better to be safe than sorry; so make sure that your phone is a safe distance away!

15) TECH-**NO**-LOGY!

Everyone does it; we get into bed, then put the TV on, have a quick look on our laptop, or have a little session on our mobile phone! This really can have a negative impact on the amount of sleep you get as well as the quality of sleep you will achieve. A study by the National Sleep Foundation found that 95% of all Americans use technology within the last hour before bed at night [9]. Using technology keeps the brain alert and as a result we can often struggle to fall asleep. If you really have to use technology before you go to bed, try dimming the brightness to lessen the effects. It would be best if you can avoid technology all together the hour or so leading up to bed time. If it is too tempting simply keep technology out of the bedroom and place this book at your bedside instead!

16) CAT NAP!

Everyone loves a good afternoon nap, especially on a Sunday, but there is a perfect time to nap as not to disrupt our evening sleep. I'm sure we have all been in the position when we slept for too long in the afternoon and now we can't drift off at night. Our alertness normally peaks around 9am and then goes downhill starting around 11am. We normally blame a heavy lunch for the tiredness but it turns out that it is natural to feel tired in the early afternoon. Our energy levels tend to hit their lowest point between 1pm and 3pm making it the PERFECT time for a nap. If you do plan to nap, try drinking a cup of coffee or caffeinated tea beforehand, this can help to increase productivity when you wake up. Coffee normally takes a while to kick in and should peak once you have woken up. So now you know how to nap and STILL sleep well in the evening. You are welcome!

17) TIRE YOURSELF OUT!

It makes sense to tire yourself during the day so you can sleep easy at night but it is something that we still don't do. If you find yourself full of energy in the early evening, it is likely that you will struggle to settle in a few hours' time. You need to find a way to expend some energy; going for a short walk is a great way to achieve this. There is NOTHING more frustrating than not being able to sleep! Think of yourself as a toddler or a high energy dog, sometimes you just need to be let out and play to burn some energy off, ha! If you still find yourself alert, take notice as to how much caffeine you are consuming (and how late in the day).

18) RELAXING SOUNDS!

Even when we are asleep, we are listening for any signs of danger. For this reason, calm and soothing noises help us to relax and eventually fall asleep (especially if you have loud noises outside your house). Natural sounds like a waterfall or the rain can help us relax into a deep sleep.

19) NIGHTLY SOAK!

Having a bath shortly before you are due to sleep is also going to help you to relax. A bath artificially raises your temperature and then it drops as soon as you get out; sending signals to your body that it is time for bed!

20) CLEAR YOUR MIND!

One of the biggest preventers of sleep is all of the thoughts that you have floating around in your mind! I'm sure you have been in the situation where you are trying to sleep but can't because your mind is racing. Maybe it is a presentation at work tomorrow or a big date with someone you like; whatever the reason, it can be a PAIN! Try writing down all of your thoughts on a piece of paper, or in a journal; this exercise will help to completely clear and calm your mind. It will be like you are actually transferring the thoughts from your mind onto the piece of paper!

21) USE YOUR BED FOR SLEEP (and maybe one other thing)!

This is one of the most common pieces of advice regarding sleep but remains SO IMPORTANT. Bedrooms should be kept solely as what they were intended for (i.e. sleeping and getting some nookie)! Sometimes, the only peace and quiet we can get in the house is our rooms so we choose to work or study in there, but this can be extremely detrimental to our sleep. As human beings, we need to completely differentiate our 'sleeping and resting area' from our 'working area'.

22) SMELLS LOVELY!

Research carried out all over the world has discovered that pleasant smells, especially lavender, make it easier for us to sleep as they enter your nostrils and send calming tones through your body. Many studies have been completed demonstrating pleasant smells help us to drift off into a natural sleep. Smells can help us recall memories and help us imagine a relaxing scenario which takes our mind off of other things.

23) A SLEEP DIVIDED!

It is perfectly normal to wake up in the middle of the night but how you deal with it is what's important! Staring at a laptop or phone screen will not help the situation and will lead to you staying up for hours. What you should do is occupy yourself for twenty to thirty minutes; maybe read a chapter of a book.....how about this book? This practice was common in pre-industrial times and they embraced it as a 'first' and 'second' sleep; they would use the time in between to read, pray, have sex (awesome!) and sometimes even visit with the neighbors!

24) EAT A KIWI!

Research suggests that kiwis not only taste great but also have significant benefits when it comes to sleep. Researchers in Taiwan tested the correlation between eating kiwis (on a daily basis) and sleep; the results suggested that the fruit improved both sleep quantity AND quality [6]!

25) GREEK YOGURT!

Greek yogurt can be extremely helpful in getting you to sleep as it contains a chemical called tryptophan which is known for its sleep inducing properties! Greek yogurt with fresh fruit could be the perfect way to get you to sleep at night! It may be a great idea to try Greek Yogurt with Kiwi (see #24 above) and some cinnamon, yum! You will get some restful sleep, healthy fats, protein, and loads of Vitamin C from the kiwi!

26) OATMEAL!

Of course, oatmeal is seen as a great option for breakfast but there are also benefits to having it before you go to bed. Amino acids, B-vitamins, and a variety of other nutrients can be found in oatmeal which are extremely effective for promoting sleep and relaxing the body!

27) LET'S GO BANANAS!

In the word of Gwen Stefani, B-A-N-A-N-A-S! As well as tasting great and being healthy, bananas have muscle relaxing properties such as potassium and magnesium along with tryptophan making them a perfect night-time snack! Sweet potatoes give the same results!

28) HUMMUS!

Chickpeas are the main ingredient in any decent hummus. Chickpeas contain vitamin B6 which is integral for the production of tryptophan, making it a great nighttime snack! Hummus is also known for its high fiber content! (Be careful with the spicy Hummus at night as spices can elevate your metabolism and keep you up longer than desired).

29) CHERRIES!

Cherries are a much sweeter option than oats and hummus but again have the same relaxing effects on our bodies. Cherries, especially tart ones, are rich in melatonin which is a sleep hormone! It is one of the few foods that contain melatonin, along with pineapples and oranges. Cherries are also a great late night snack that is low glycemic and won't spike your blood sugar levels; as elevated blood sugar levels lead to fat storage. Cherries can also decrease inflammation and help repair tissue.

30) STAY COMFORTABLE!

Your body has to be at a comfortable temperature to fall asleep, so you will struggle if you are too hot or too cold! Keeping our bedroom at the right temperature will place us in a much better position to drift off! If you are too cold, a great option is spooning; I know my wife loves being 'little spoon' when she is cold since I'm a human heat source…..although, when I'm cold I'm not ashamed to say I like to be 'little spoon' from time to time.

31) SLEEP NAKED!

When I tell people to sleep naked, they often give me a look of disapproval; however, when I explain the benefits they are EXTREMELY grateful in a few weeks' time (both them and their significant others)! After reading this, you will never sleep with ANY clothing on again! Sleeping naked improves quality and quantity of sleep, reduces stress, blood pressure and cholesterol, can keep you looking young, and can improve your sex life!

✓ **IMPROVED QUALITY AND QUANTITY!** – Sleeping naked is proven to help both the amount of sleep we get and to which extent that sleep is achieved. If we sleep naked, we are more likely to reach a deeper sleep and stay in those deeper sleep phases for longer than if we were to have clothes on. This is because our body temperature is regulated in a more efficient way; we are able to reach the correct temperature and stay there for longer. The blanket on top of the sheets can even sometimes have an effect as they keep us warm (sometimes too warm) and tend to make us uncomfortable!

✓ **REDUCE STRESS, BLOOD PRESSURE AND CHOLESTEROL!** – 'How on earth?' But it is completely true! It is again related to our body temperature when sleeping. As we cool, we are able to lower our cortisol level, which is also known as the 'stress hormone.' Reducing cortisol can lead to a number of health benefits including reduced blood pressure, better cholesterol levels, better sleep, appetite regulation, reduced stress levels, as well as improve our immune system!

- ✓ **BEAUTY SLEEP!** – Melatonin and growth hormones are the two most important anti-aging hormones in our body and these can be limited when we are too hot in our sleep. It is believed that sleeping in a bedroom hotter than 69.8 degrees Fahrenheit will prevent them from being released altogether! Furthermore, both hormones need cool temperatures as well as darkness in order to be released! Sleeping naked is starting to look like a good option now, isn't it?

- ✓ **ITS ALL ABOUT THE NOOKIE!** – This tip may just be the one that persuades you to finally strip off when it comes to bed time, and there is scientific evidence to back it up! There is a powerful hormone called oxytocin, otherwise known as the love hormone; I think this is what Cupid puts on his arrows. Oxytocin can be released due to skin-to-skin contact with your partner. Oxytocin is responsible for orgasms and sexual responsiveness, blood pressure reduction, combating stress and depression, and reducing intestinal inflammation! Plus sleeping naked next to each other is more often than not enough to get people going anyway!

If these GREAT benefits aren't enough to get you in your birthday suit tonight then I don't know what is! Ooh, maybe this will put you over the edge…there is also evidence that shows sleeping naked can help lower your body fat! Get skinny while you sleep? Yes please! So why not give it a go tonight?

32) SLEEP COLD TO GET LEAN!

Sleeping in a room of a temperature of 66 degrees was shown to increase the amount of brown fat (good metabolically active fat) in our bodies! Having more brown fat increases our fat burning potential of the nasty white fat we don't want as well as gets rid of excess blood sugar [18]! Originally, scientists thought that babies only had brown fat but it has been discovered that adults have brown fat as well. In fact, according to a 2014 study carried out by the National Institutes of Health, sleeping in a cold room can help boost your metabolism [4]! So if you want to get a restful sleep and leaner turn down your thermostat to 66 degrees. If that's too cold for you its ok, even a small temperature decrease has been shown to have slight calorie burning benefits. Now get some LEAN ZZZZ's!

33) ALARM GOES OFF, LIGHTS GO ON!

This tip can be particularly handy if you struggle to wake up in the morning (even after setting several alarms on your phone). As soon as your alarm goes off, throw the lights on to let your body know you are getting up! Trying to wake up in the dark can be difficult because it is so tempting to press the snooze button and slide back under the covers!

34) MORNING ALARM!

Make sure you have the alarm clock out of arms reach so you can't press the snooze button in the morning! You are more likely to get up and get on with the day if you have to get out of bed to turn the alarm off!

THE FOUNDATION: NUTRITION

In this section, we are going to take a look at some of the great hacks out there in regards to nutrition. When attempting to lose weight, our diet is one of THE MOST important things to consider. It is easy to think 'I am doing my part by exercising, so I don't have to worry about what I eat' or 'I have just gone for a run so that means I can have a chocolate bar as a treat'; however, this couldn't be further from the truth. Ever heard the saying 'abs are made in the kitchen and not in the gym?' Yup, that's right. You CANNOT out work bad eating habits! It is now thought that nearly 40% of Americans are obese; 40%! This is up from 32% in 2004! At the same time, it is thought that our nutritional options HAVE IMPROVED so why are we getting fatter? Lack of education! People are unaware of the fantastic foods available to them; they are unaware of exactly what they need to eat to stay healthy and why they need it! ONE IN FOUR Americans say that they consume LESS than one serving of vegetables a day; just think about how much processed 'crap' food makes its way into our daily meals! If you are serious about losing weight and making a change to your life then you have to pay attention to what you eat.

Before I get into the hacks of nutrition, let's start with a little science refresher, the basics of nutrition. Nutrition regards the composition of foods and beverages required to sustain life, provide energy, and prevent poor health or disease. We refer to it as nutrition because it is designed to nourish us; in addition to providing our daily caloric needs. As I mentioned before, we are a nation that is overfed and undernourished. We have to move away from the mentality of eating for calories (and way too many mind you) and move towards the mentality of meeting both our caloric and nutrient requirements.

Many of us have heard the old saying 'you are what you eat', which rings true to a large extent. Food is not only the fuel used by your body, it is also the building material of the structure of your body; much like building materials required for a house. Your diet, including beverages and supplements, not only provides you with energy, but helps to form the structure of your cells, creates your biochemistry, affects alertness and mood, and may cause or prevent sickness and disease. We all know that we have to use the proper oil and fuel in our vehicles in order for it to run efficiently. Think of your nutrients as the oil and calories as fuel for your body. Just like improper maintenance will ruin your vehicle; prolonged nutritional deprivation (or caloric overload) will wreak havoc to your health.

In my opinion there is NOTHING more important than the composition of your diet when it comes to your health and appearance, even MORE important than exercise. Yes, I said it, what you eat is MORE important to your health over exercise! I would go so far as to say, many of the lifestyle diseases which affect such a large number of people in Western society could be prevented by the consumption of healthier foods and beverages. According to the CDC our number one killer in this country is lifestyle related; heart disease kills over 610,000 (1 in 4) Americans EVERY year [16]! No matter how much or how hard you train, if your effort is not supported by good food and beverage choices, you will not be able to reap the health benefits of your hard work.

Your diet is comprised of five major nutrients placed within two categories. The macronutrients are carbohydrates, protein, and fats. The micronutrients are vitamins and minerals. All are required in the diet. The required amounts of each will vary according to your needs. A larger man requires more than a smaller man. A more active female requires more than a less active female. Building muscular size requires more calories than losing size or shedding body fat. Heavy training requires a diet which supports not only the activity of the program itself, but also supports the recovery process and muscular growth (hypertrophy).

Carbohydrates provide the largest portion of most diets in terms of volume. It provides a little over 4 calories per gram. Carbohydrates are required for energy, blood sugar regulation, and it is the body's (including the brain's) preferred source of fuel. You NEED carbohydrates to survive, and depending on your goals you may need a higher carbohydrate intake, a lower carbohydrate intake, or a combination of both (i.e. cycling carbohydrates when trying to lose body fat (refer to hack #50)). All carbohydrates get broken down into simple sugar. In the blood stream, its form is blood sugar, in the muscles and liver, its storage form is glycogen. It is used efficiently by the body and most of us have cravings for carbohydrate foods due to the energy release and mood boosting effects they provide. However, overconsumption of carbohydrates, especially in refined or processed form, can cause major health problems; it can elevate blood sugar levels causing the pancreas to release insulin. In smaller amounts, it presents little issue. In larger amounts, it may be a precursor to weight gain, insulin resistance, future diabetes, and perhaps heart disease.

Carbohydrates are chains of saccharides (sugars), some are simpler, others more complex; all of which are broken down during digestion into their simplest form, glucose. For our purpose, we will draw the main distinction between refined and unrefined carbohydrates.

✓ **Refined carbohydrates** are processed and include sweets, sodas, crackers, breads etc. During processing; fiber, vitamins, and minerals are stripped from the carbohydrates. What is left is a "food like substance" which still has calories, but lacks most, if not all, of the nutritional value it originally contained. These carbohydrates typically have a high glycemic index; the rate at which a carbohydrate food is broken down into blood sugar. I want you to LIMIT these refined carbohydrate foods. From my perspective they have little to no value as a nutritional substance, and will not support your efforts to build a healthy, muscular, and lean physique.

✓ **Unrefined carbohydrates** do not go through the refinement process. As such, they are more complex food substances with higher nutritional value. Typically they have more fiber, more vitamins and minerals, and a lower glycemic index. This includes fruits, vegetables, quinoa, wild and brown rice, coarse breads with very few ingredients, whole grain pastas, etc. I want you to get your carbohydrates from this group. These foods are great for you, providing large quantities of more complex sugars, fiber, vitamins, minerals, and water. As lower glycemic carbohydrate foods, they will release a more steady supply of energy to your body and your brain; allowing you to function more efficiently for longer periods of time. That is exactly what you want. Make sure that you consume moderate to high quantities of these foods, depending on your ultimate goal.

Protein yields a little over four calories per gram. Amino acids are contained within polypeptides, which are chains of molecules. Nine are essential, which means that they must be ingested in the diet. Twelve are nonessential, which means that they can be produced within the body.

When building muscle, protein is essential to your diet. It is required for tissue repair and growth, which stimulates hypertrophy, or muscle gain. It has been the staple of athletes and strongmen for centuries, dating back to days of ancient Greece in which strongmen such as Milos would consume large quantities. It was believed that consumption of flesh and other animal products contributed to strength and muscle gain and such knowledge remains true.

I recommend getting your protein requirements through lean meats, fish, poultry, eggs, dairy, nuts, beans, seeds, and engineered protein foods such as whey protein powder. As with carbohydrates, I would prefer that your animal protein comes from foods which are organic or unprocessed. Regular supplies of beef, pork, lamb, chicken, turkey, etc. may come from animals which have been hormone fed to stimulate rapid gains in size and maturity. They may also have been fed an inferior diet of genetically modified corns and grains, rather than grass and other natural feed sources.

Vegetarians and vegans may get protein in their diets through nuts, seeds, grains, and legumes, but food combining is necessary to create complete proteins; which mean that the full complement of amino acids is present in the diet. If you are in this category, I recommend that you consult with a nutritionist or dietician to make sure that you are not amino acid deficient.

Fats consist of a group of compounds which are generally insoluble in water. In chemical form, they are triglycerides of glycerol and fatty acids. Fats may be solid or liquid at room temperature, depending on structure and composition. Fats (a.k.a lipids and oils) are important to all animals, including humans, serving structural and metabolic functions. Fats have the highest energy yield of all macronutrients at just over 9 calories per gram, compared to a little over 4 calories per gram for both carbohydrates and protein. Though not generally used as efficiently by the body as carbohydrates, they are an important component of the diet and should not under any circumstances be eliminated completely. Fats support a number of the body's functions, and some vitamins must have fat to dissolve and nourish your body.

There is however, a less desirable aspect to the consumption of fats. The concern with some types of fat, and its cousin cholesterol, is that it may play a role in cardiovascular disease and Type 2 diabetes. Dietary fats may also play a role in other diseases, such as obesity and cancer; although evidence is mounting that it often occurs in the presence of overconsumption of processed carbohydrates. Research about the potential harmful effects of dietary fats is evolving, and suggests that you should focus on consuming healthy fats and avoid unhealthy fats.

The two types of healthy dietary fats are monounsaturated fat and polyunsaturated fat.

- ✓ **Monounsaturated fat** is found in a variety of foods and oils. Studies suggest that eating foods rich in monounsaturated fats improves blood cholesterol levels, which may decrease your risk of heart disease. Research also suggests that monounsaturated fats may benefit insulin levels and blood sugar control, which is particularly helpful in the case of Type 2 diabetes.

- ✓ **Polyunsaturated fat** is found mainly in plant based foods and oils. Research suggests that eating foods rich in polyunsaturated fats improves blood cholesterols, which decrease the risk of Type 2 diabetes. One type of polyunsaturated fat in particular, omega-3 fatty acids may be especially beneficial to the heart. These fats, found in fatty fish, appear to decrease the risk of coronary disease. They may also protect against irregular heartbeats and help lower blood pressure levels. Foods made up of mostly monounsaturated and polyunsaturated fats are liquid at room temperature, such as olive oil, avocado oil, and grapeseed oil.

The two main types of potentially harmful dietary fat are saturated fat and trans fat. Most fats which have a high percentage of saturated fat or trans fat are solid at room temperature. Because of this property, they are usually referred to as solid fats. They include pork fat, beef fat, margarine, butter, and shortening.

- ✓ **Saturated fat** mainly comes from animal sources and raises total blood cholesterol levels and low-density lipoprotein (LDL) cholesterol levels, which may increase the risk of cardiovascular disease; although more and more research is pointing to sugar and refined carbs being more of a problem than saturated fats. In general, foods with saturated fat are higher in calories and may contribute to increased risk of Type 2 diabetes and heart disease. Some saturated fat is ok, especially coconut oil, just limit your consumption of unhealthy saturated fats and replace with other healthy polyunsaturated fats when possible.

✓ **Trans fat** occurs naturally in some foods, especially those from animals. Most however, are made during food processing through partial hydrogenation of unsaturated fats. This process creates fats which are easier to cook with and less likely to spoil than naturally occurring oils. These trans fats are also called industrial or synthetic trans fats. Research suggests that these trans fats can increase unhealthy LDL cholesterol and lower healthy high-density lipoprotein (HDL) cholesterol. This may increase your risk of cardiovascular disease.

Cholesterol, often thought of as a fat, is not a fat, but rather a waxy, fat like substance. Our bodies manufacture some, but also absorb dietary cholesterol, found in foods derived from animal sources. It is a vital substance because it builds cells in the body and produces hormones. However, our bodies produce enough so we do not need it through dietary intake. Excessive cholesterol in the diet can increase your unhealthy LDL cholesterol levels. This may lead to heart disease and stroke. Most foods which contain saturated fat also contain cholesterol, so cutting back on these foods will decrease the intake of both. Tropical oils such as coconut oils are an exception to this, containing saturated fat, but not cholesterol.

Vitamins and minerals (the micronutrients) are also an essential component of nutrition. There is far too much information for me to go into detail here and I don't want to bore you, "JUST GIVE ME THE HACKS JOEY!" I will touch on just a few of the main ones, and why they are important to you. Most vitamins and minerals will be ingested with your foods and beverages; however, if your diet provides insufficient amounts, supplementation will be important to you. My preference is always to derive vitamins and minerals through natural food and beverage products, although I do support supplementation with certain products.

Vitamins are organic substances (made by plants or animals), whereas minerals are inorganic substances which come from the earth, soil and water, and are absorbed by plants. Animals and humans absorb minerals from the plants they eat. Vitamins and minerals are nutrients required by the body for normal growth and development.

There are **13 vitamins** which our bodies need to grow and develop normally. They are A, C, D, E, K and the B vitamins (thiamine, riboflavin, niacin, pantothenic acid, biotin, vitamin B-6, vitamin B-12 and folate). As suggested, virtually all of these will come from the foods you eat. Your body is also able to make vitamin D and K. Vegetarians may need to take a vitamin B-12 supplement. Each vitamin has a specific job. If you are deficient in certain vitamins, you may develop a deficiency disease. Inadequate vitamin D for example, may cause rickets and lack of vitamin C may cause scurvy. Some vitamins also prevent medical problems (vitamin A prevents night blindness). The best way to get enough vitamins is to eat a balanced, nutritious diet with a variety of healthy, natural foods. In some cases, a multivitamin may be taken for optimal health. High doses of some vitamins can make you sick.

Minerals are also important for your body to stay healthy. Your body uses minerals for many different jobs, including building bones, making hormones, and regulating heartbeat.

There are 2 kinds of minerals: macro minerals and trace minerals. Macro minerals are required by your body in larger amounts. They include calcium, phosphorus, magnesium, sodium, potassium, chloride, and sulfur. Your body needs only small amounts of trace minerals, which include iron, manganese, copper, iodine, zinc, cobalt, fluoride, and selenium.

As with vitamins, the best way to get the minerals your body requires is by eating a large variety of healthy, natural foods. If deficient, your doctor may recommend a mineral supplement.

Water is essential to life on our planet. You are no exception. Our bodies are comprised of almost 70% water, which causes cells to have structure and function. Without it, we would die in a few days. Besides allowing cells and organs to function, water serves as a lubricant in the body, making up saliva and the fluids surrounding the joints. Water regulates body temperature through perspiration. It also helps to prevent and relieve constipation by moving foods through the intestines.

We derive some of the water in our bodies through the foods we eat. Some water is made through the process of metabolism. Drinking water, however, is our main and best source of water ingestion. We may also get water through the consumption of liquid foods and beverages such as milk, soup, or juices. However, beverages containing caffeine such as coffee, tea, soda, and alcoholic beverages have a diuretic effect (cause the body to excrete water) and are therefore not the best choices for your water consumption. The side effects of not drinking enough water can be severe, and even deadly if it persists for long enough. Dehydration (caused by too little water ingestion) will cause the body's fluids to be out of balance, leading to other health complications.

Below, I am going to tell you EXACTLY why junk food is so bad for you and what they do to your body and then onto some great nutrition 'tips and hacks' to set you on the right path!

Why Is Junk Food So Bad?

We have been hearing it for so long, 'stay away from junk food!' 'It isn't good for you' but not many people know the full extent of how damaging it could be to our bodies and now is the time to learn! Once you have finished reading this section, you will want to stay away from all junk foods for a long time (that's the idea anyway!). Keep this statement in your head, if you eat junk, you will feel and look like junk!

Nowadays, with the rise of 'ready-meals' and other similar products, it is easy to consistently get a sufficient amount of calories, but calories aren't everything! What you don't get in these meals are key nutrients and minerals. It is thought that within just FIVE DAYS of eating junk food, your muscles start struggling to oxidize glucose (the storage form of carbs). Normally, your muscles will either break down the glucose or store it for a later date; and muscles make up about 30% of our total body weight. If you were to lose muscle tissue this can be severely damaging to your health and lead to a large list of problems including diabetes.

I quite often hear 'well, one meal won't make a difference' or even 'a couple of unhealthy days won't affect me' when this is completely untrue! We are putting ourselves in danger of a plethora of health problems with EACH AND EVERY piece of junk food we consume. In the long-term, the spike in sugar levels we receive after an unhealthy meal can cause 'post-prandial hyperglycemia (dramatic rise in blood sugar following a meal)' which can ultimately increase the chances of getting cancer. However, we also experience many short-term problems such as; inflamed tissue (just as we get with infection), constricting blood vessels and high blood pressure. The surge and the dramatic drop you receive in insulin may also cause you to feel hungry soon after the meal which may lead to further unhealthy eating as your day progresses.

Have you ever had a high carb and/or sugar meal and literally couldn't control your appetite? You NEED another cookie, and another, and another....I know. I have also had this feeling and there is a chemical reason for this; you have triggered your reptilian response part of your brain that craves junk! This response in your body is muck like a drug addict needing more drugs to get his fix. So basically your reaction to sweets and crap food at that moment is that of a cocaine addict needing another bump...yes, I just compared eating junk food to an addict because sugar is now your FIX! It is often said that our health is as good as our last meal so a healthy meal may help to return our bodies back to their normal state. However, that doesn't remove what it has been through. It also doesn't remove the long-term damage that may have been caused.

Junk food also puts A LOT of unnecessary stress on our digestive system, which is now working overtime to break down the high processed foods that are in our systems. If a food sits for a long time in our digestive tract and it's nutritionally dense our bodies can eventually break down that food and still absorb all the nutrients within. When it comes to junk food (this is why they are EMPTY calories), it means that all the nasties stay in our system for longer (often in the form of fat) and we don't receive any benefit from it whatsoever, in fact, it is more likely to cause damage!

It is thought that people who consume more instant noodles, for example, are at a greater risk of metabolic syndrome (increased BP, high blood sugar levels, excess abdominal fat, and increased risk of heart disease, stroke, and diabetes) than those who eat less, REGARDLESS OF OVERALL DIET OR EXERCISE! You also have to remember what we feed our microbiome as well as ourselves can have a HUGE effect on our future ('gut health' protects us against germs, breaks down food for energy, and produces vitamins). If we are constantly giving our digestive system junk food, we may be altering the way it is set up and this can affect MANY biological processes including our memory. If we don't look after it, we may end up risking not only our health but also our well-being!

Obesity is now thought to be more dangerous than smoking! Just think about that for a second; we have reached a point in time where more doctors' visits are linked to obesity than tobacco use. The global cost of obesity has now hit $2 TRILLION which is level with smoking and armed violence. Yet, despite these horrifying statistics, the problem still isn't being taken seriously enough! Luckily for you though, you have purchased this book and are paving the way towards a brighter future.

Nutrition Hacks

35) JUST SAY NO TO BULLIES!

Before we get started, you need to get used to saying the word 'no'! Say it now! Say it aloud, shout it if you want to; three times! NO, NO, NO! Now, this isn't necessarily just about saying no to unhealthy foods, this is about saying no to people who are trying to get you to eat unhealthily. Of course, we should try to remove all negativity from our lives but even the positive people may still try and get us to go against our diet; but we are NOT having it! Who would've thought when we became adults (at least in age) that we would still run into bullies! People want to get us to be like them and try to bully us into eating bad! Instead of saying I want that but I can't eat it, change your mindset and say **I CAN HAVE THAT, but I DON'T WANT IT!** Maybe a family member is trying to get you to have a second slice of dessert or more than one glass of wine, tell them 'no' and then move on. Once you let them know that you are strong and you will not be folding, they will soon back down and no longer ask. Just say NO!

36) KNOW YOUR EXACT METABOLIC NEEDS!

Ever wondered EXACTLY how many calories your body burns in a day and how many calories you need to gain or lose weight? Well your Basal Metabolic Rate (BMR) is the minimum level of energy required to maintain the body's vital functions in a waking state. So once you know your BMR you can figure out EXACTLY what your macronutrient and caloric intake should be to reach your desired health goal.

Determine your BMR following this simple formula developed by Dr. Fred Hatfield based on your bodyweight in kg (1kg = 2.2lbs).

Men BMR = 1x (bodyweight in kg) x 24
Women BMR = .9 x (bodyweight in kg) x 24

Here's an example: (remember, this is only an example and you will need to substitute your weight in kg and specific activity level for each calculation)

If you are a 175 pound male: 175 pounds/2.2 = 79.5kg.
Your BMR formula is: 1 x (79.5 x 24) = 1908 calories

Note: The formula is for bodyweight and not lean body mass. It will be accurate if you are in the normal body fat range of 14-19% for men and 20-25% for women. If you are above these ranges, the formula will OVERESTIMATE your calories and you will need to figure out your BMR based on the following formula:

BMR (for men and women) = 370 + (21.6 x lean mass in kg)

If you know your body fat percentage, use this formula also, as it is slightly more accurate

(lean mass = your weight - pounds of fat)

Total Daily Energy Expenditure

Now that you know your BMR, you can determine your TDEE, or Total Daily Energy Expenditure, which is the number of calories required to maintain your current weight.

To get your TDEE, you must first figure out you activity factor:

> **Sedentary:** workout 0-1 times per week: multiply your BMR by 1.2
>
> **Lightly active:** workout 1-2 times per week: multiply your BMR by 1.375
>
> **Moderately active:** workout 3-4 times per week: multiply your BMR by 1.55
>
> **Very active:** workout 4-5 times per week: multiply your BMR by 1.725
>
> **Extremely active:** workout 6-7 times per week: multiply your BMR by 1.9

So, continuing with the example, if you are a moderately active 175 pound (79.5kg) male with a BMR of 1,908. TDEE = 1,908 x 1.55 = 2,957 calories

Here try it out for yourself:

> Your weight in kilograms _____ (your weight in pounds / 2.2)
>
> Your BMR _____
>
> (For men: 1 x your weight in kg x 24)
>
> (For women:0 .9 x your weight in kg x 24)
>
> Your TDEE _____ (BMR x your activity factor)

37) BAD CALORIE VS. GOOD CALORIE!

Do you really think if you eat 1,000 calories of vegetables that it is exactly the same for your body as consuming two candy bars?! Absolutely not! The only thing that a calorie in a candy bar and a calorie from a vegetable have in common is that they contain the same amount of energy. One dietary calorie contains 4,184 Joules of energy. In that respect, then yes, a calorie is a calorie.

However when it comes to your body, things are not that cut and dry. The human body is a complex system with elaborate processes that regulate energy balance. Different foods are processed differently by the body; some are inefficient and cause energy (calories) to be lost as heat [36]. Different foods and macronutrients can affect the way we feel, our metabolism, and even determine our hunger levels.

Here are some sound examples of how each calorie is unique:

✓ **Fructose and Glucose:** There are two main simple sugars in the foods we eat known as fructose and glucose. Both of these have similar chemical structures but they behave differently once they begin to be digested within our systems. Glucose can be metabolized by all of the body's tissues, but fructose can only be metabolized by the liver. Before you get upset with me and say, Joey, fructose is in fruit so it's good for me! I'm only talking about fructose from added sugars, not real fruit which has vitamins, nutrients, and fiber to slow down the digestion. Here's why fructose and glucose differ:

> ✓ Fructose does not satisfy the brain's satiety center as well as glucose does (you don't feel as full).
>
> ✓ Our hunger hormone known as Ghrelin goes up when we're hungry and should go down after we eat. Fructose can lead to higher hunger levels when eaten as opposed to glucose [37].
>
> ✓ High amounts of fructose can cause insulin resistance (due to a spiked blood sugar level), stomach fat gain, increased triglycerides, and elevated LDL (bad) cholesterol compared to the same number of calories from glucose [39].

✓ **Thermic Effect of Food (TEF):** As discussed more in depth in hack #47, certain foods can elevate the metabolism more than others. Eating lean protein will burn more calories than fat or carbs. Whole foods simply require more energy to digest than 'food-like' substances.

✓ **Different foods have different effects on our hunger levels.** If you are to eat foods that are high in processed sugars you aren't going to be as satisfied as you would be if you were to eat a food that is high in nutrients like vegetables, fruit, and protein. Protein is one of the highest satiating foods that you can eat.

✓ **Glycemic Index:** Talk to 10 different health professionals and you will probably get 10 different answers on what someone should eat. But a general consensus is that refined carbohydrates need to be avoided! These are nutritionally hollow, have low fiber, are highly processed, and get digested incredibly quickly by the body leading to a rapid spike in blood sugar, hunger levels, and fat storage. When we eat these processed carbs we have what is called a neuropeptide Y (NPY) response in the hypothalamus and causes us to overeat uncontrollably [38]. This response is much like a drug addict.

As you can see calories matter, but more often than not it is what you eat that can have the biggest effect on your body, hormones, and potential overeating!

38) KNOW YOUR MACROS!

Now that you know how many calories you have to eat to maintain, gain, or lose weight (refer to hack #36), you are all set right? Wrong! It irks me when people think all they have to do is eat 'X' amount of calories to reach their goals because they believe a calorie is just a calorie. Now you know better (refer to hack #37). Sure, you can lose weight lowering your overall calories but if you eat the wrong food you could risk losing bone density, losing too much muscle tissue as opposed to fat, and lowering your metabolism. The same goes if you want to maintain your weight or gain muscle; eating nutrient dense calories will pack on the muscle, not fat!

39) KNOW YOUR MACRO RATIO!

There are so many diets out there from low carb to high carb, low fat to high fat, the cookie diet (that was actually a thing), and everything in between. Here are a few factors that you should include when deciding what your diet should be:

- ✓ Establish your goals (refer to hack #3) - Do you want to lose fat, maintain your weight, or build muscle?

- ✓ Figure out your TDEE and calories (refer to hack #36)

- ✓ Know your **Body Type** (refer to hack #40)

- ✓ General percentage (ratio) of calories in your diet that you need for your goals:

    - ✓ **Lose Fat** (Lower Carb): 15-30% Carbs, Fat 25-35%, Protein 35-50%

    - ✓ **Maintain** (Moderate Carb): 30-50% Carbs, Fat 25-35%, Protein 25-35%

    - ✓ **Build Muscle** (High Carb): 40-60% Carbs, Fat 15-25%, Protein 25-35%

Remember when calculating your macros simply multiply your daily calorie needs by the percentage and that will give you how many calories you need of each macronutrient.

Now there are obvious variations to these ranges but sticking with these for a few weeks and tracking your progress is a great way to really dial in on your nutrition. Dietary fat doesn't drop below 15% in any range no matter what your goal is. Besides us needing fat to survive, fat also regulates our hormones like testosterone and estrogen (amongst others) that can affect your mood, reproduction, growth hormone development, metabolism, and the absorption of vitamins A, D, E, and K. Even more severe, not getting enough essential fatty acids can increase the risk of several cancers including breast, prostate, and colon.

40) KNOW YOUR BODY TYPE!

I'm 'big boned.' 'I have a slow metabolism.' 'I look like a pear.' 'I add muscle too fast and get bulky!' These are all related to one thing; what type of body you have. In other words, the way you look, how you store fat, process carbohydrates, and add muscle can help determine what your macronutrients should be. There are three 'main' types of bodies, but we all know life isn't so black and white. It is common to fall into more than one category.

The THREE body types are (for our purposes we are going to focus on body type and carbohydrate percentages; the other remainder of the calories will come from protein and fat):

✓ **Ectomorph:** You are a slender individual with narrow shoulders and frame. Your metabolism is incredibly high and growing up you may have been called Gumby; ok, maybe that was just me! This is often called a 'hard gainer' since it's very hard to put on muscle and/or fat. Ectomorphs respond well to a higher range of carbohydrates between 30-60% of total calories. If you fall into this category and want to maintain weight, 45-50% of your calories should come from carbohydrates. If your goal is to gain mass, stick to the high range of carbs (55-60%). If you want to lose weight stick to 25-30% for carbohydrate intake.

✓ **Mesomorph** is someone who tends to put on muscle easily; they are very strong, athletic, and have a hard dense muscular structure. Often people who grow up playing sports that require lots of strength and sprinting are meso-morph due to the training demand on their muscular system. Mesomorphs can generally lose fat fast and gain muscle, but will put on fat faster than an ectomorph. Mesomorphs are able to store muscle glycogen (storage form of carbs in the muscle); in turn they usually handle carbs well and utilize them for energy. Total calories from carbs should be 20-50%. Mesomorphs should stay within the middle to high range for all ratios. Fat loss 20-30% of calories, for weight maintenance carbs are 40-50% of calories, and for muscle gain stick to 50-60%.

✓ **Endomorph:** This is best described as someone who is soft in the mid-dle, holds on to fat easily, is generally stocky or shorter in build, has a slow metabolism, has narrow shoulders and wide lower body; or 'pear shaped'. Endomorph's are able to put on a decent amount of muscle but also carry more fat as excess carbohydrates (especially refined) that can cause you to gain weight. Endomorphs should stay within the lower carbohydrate range for all of your goals, between 10-40 percent of total calories. I recom-mend 10-20% for fat loss, 20-30% for maintenance, and 40-50% carbs for mass gains.

41) CUT 200-300 CALORIES NOT 500!

In 1958 scientist Max Wishnofsky concluded that the caloric equivalent of one pound loss or gain of bodyweight was equal to 3500 calories. Ever since, this has become the gold standard for how many calories we need to cut or add to gain or lose a pound of fat. So if you were to cut 500 calories a day for 52 weeks you would, in theory, lose 52 pounds; the equivalent of a small child, awesome! Now one thing people don't tell you is that the body is incredibly resilient to any changes in diet. These 52 pounds is a gross OVER estimate of the amount of weight which can be lost by reducing your cal-orie intake. When you reduce your calorie intake your body responds by making you burn fewer calories. Your body becomes more efficient at doing the same amount of work with fewer calories than before...bummer!! Now the solution to this problem is to slowly cut your calories (ideally cut the sugar and processed foods out first). By cut-ting 200-300 calories a day (as opposed to 500) for a week or two and see your results. You may also exercise (highly recommended) which will increase your calorie burn at the same time. Do this until the scale seems to plateau and then cut more calories from your diet (about 20-25% of your total TDEE) and/or MOVE more, plain and simple! Once you know exactly how many calories you burn in a day you can start by subtracting or adding calories based on your desired goals.

42) FRONT LOAD YOUR CALORIES!

Now that you know exactly how many calories you need in a day you can really dial in on your nutrition and get your body on the correct health path! So what does FRONT LOADING your calories mean? Our metabolism slows down throughout the day and this is why we are told not to eat late at night. If we are using less energy at night and eating our largest meal at night, our bodies are less likely to utilize those calories as energy and more likely store them as fat. The solution; front load your calories. This simply means having your bigger meal earlier in the day. For example, if you are on a 2,000 calorie diet you may have 600 calories for breakfast, 300 calories for a snack, 500 calories for lunch, 200 calories for an afternoon snack, and 400 calories for dinner. Doing this will make sure the biggest meals are in the earlier part of the day so that those calories are more likely used as energy as opposed to being stored as fat. Don't worry if you don't have time for a large breakfast. I get it. Some people can barely get dressed in the morning let alone make breakfast (although there are several tips in this book to facilitate the process). Just make your lunch bigger than normal and taper down from there. Doing this will have you on a lean and healthy path in no time!

43) GET FAT!

Get fat in your diet! If you want to lose weight, get ripped, or even build muscle, cutting out dietary fat is NOT a good idea! Gone are the days of low fat and fat free diets! All that was accomplished was substituting sugar for fat, making us store more fat, thus making us fatter. Eating FAT can actually help you LOSE FAT! Why? We have "old" fat stored in our body's peripheral tissues (also called subcutaneous fat) in the stomach, butt, and thighs which can't be burned off efficiently without new dietary fat to help the process. According to researchers at Washington University School of Medicine in St. Louis, dietary fat helps break down existing fat by activating PPAR-alpha and fat-burning pathways through the liver. So eating fat will burn our stubborn stored fat! Besides helping to burn fat, eating fat helps keep us full, helps increase muscle mass, helps the absorption of fat soluble vitamins like A,C,E, and K, and has even been shown to make you happier!

But before you reach for that candy bar, it's important to eat the right kind of fat in order to reap the benefits. Good sources of omega-3 fats include: salmon, trout, sardines, walnuts and flaxseeds. Olive oil, peanuts/peanut butter, avocados, nuts, sunflower seeds, and eggs, yes, the entire egg (refer to hack #86) are all good sources of monounsaturated fats. Keep your fat intake to 15-35% of your calories.

44) EAT SLOW DIGESTING CARBS!

If you want to get healthy, stay healthy, provide your body with energy, and/or limit water gain make the carbs you ingest slow digesting ones. These carbs should be your first choice for fuel as they are not manufactured and loaded with lots of fiber and nutrients to produce a slow increase in blood glucose and a modest insulin release limiting the fat gaining potential. Slow digesting carbs include but not limited to: sweet potatoes, yams, wild rice, quinoa, beans, red potatoes, and fruits.

45) SAY NO TO DRUGS!

What?! I'm talking about refined sugar and processed carbohydrates. Refined sugar is rapidly digested by our systems as opposed to complex carbohydrates. For the most part the more processing involved in producing a carb, the faster it digests and turns into sugar. Foods like bagels, dinner rolls, white bread, white rice, mashed potatoes, fat-free muffins (lots of fat free foods add sugar), candy (obviously), cold cereals, rice cakes and fruit juices require one or more processing steps to manufacture; creating an environment for the carbohydrate to hit the bloodstream quicker than slow-digesting carbs. This causes an insulin spike (blood sugar goes up) creating an environment that is undesirable for most individuals resulting in a high potential for fat gain and can lead to metabolic problems such as insulin resistance and diabetes. There is one exception where you may want to have these foods…..really Joey when?….see hack #213.

46) EAT OFTEN!

Some people are perfectly fine (and capable) eating 3 clean, well-balanced and healthy meals a day with minimal snacking in between, but for others this may be difficult to achieve. One thing that I find works well with people is eating 5-6 smaller meals per day, spaced 2-3 hours apart. This allows you to stay full throughout the day and not overeat. The idea behind eating several times a day increases your metabolism is based on the fact that simply eating (chewing and digesting) food burns calories (see next hack).

47) CHEW YOUR FOOD!

There are a number of benefits from juicing and drinking smoothies, but one thing that these things don't do is actually increase your calorie burn of the food you are consuming (drinking) because your system doesn't have to process it by breaking it down. When you eat (chew) food (carbs, proteins, and fats), your body must expend energy (calories) to digest, absorb, and store the nutrients in the food you've eaten. This is called the Thermic Effect of Food (TEF) that occurs after ingestion. Simply by consuming calories you actually increase the rate at which your body burns calories. So how many calories do you burn by actually eating food? Protein is king! Your body expends more energy (calories) to process proteins than carbohydrates or fats. You'll burn up to 30 percent of the calories in lean-protein foods just by having to process them. Carbohydrates come in second with TEF average between 15 and 20 percent of the calories. The easiest digested are fats, which have a TEF of only 2 to 3 percent, (and fats have the highest calorie content as well). As a general rule you can say about 10-15% of your overall food calories will be burned through TEF. In other words if you have a 2,000 calorie diet you will burn about 200-300 calories per day from the act of eating, making your net calories for the day around 1700-1800 calories.

48) CONSIDER FASTING OVER FEASTING!

This isn't for everyone, but that's exactly what this book is about, letting you figure out tools to make your life healthier! People have been fasting for years now from personal preferences to religious reasons but we haven't had much research to back it up until recently! Intermittent Fasting (I.F.) is known as going through periods of not eating for 14-18 hours (sometimes more) followed by an eating window of generally 6-10 hours. Here's the science and the benefits behind intermittent fasting [27]:

✓ Helps promote insulin sensitivity – Optimal insulin sensitivity is crucial for your health; as insulin resistance or poor insulin sensitivity contributes to nearly all chronic diseases.

✓ Normalizes your hunger levels known as ghrelin hormone levels. Research points to a much lower need to over indulge in 'crap food' once your body adapts to the fast and turns to fat burning.

✓ Increases the rate of HGH (Human Growth Hormone) production known as the 'Fitness Hormone". Research in 2011 from the American College of Cardiology in New Orleans showed a 1,300 percent rise of HGH in women and a 2,000 percent increase in men. This has an important role in health, fitness, muscle growth, increased fat loss (without muscle loss) increased metabolism, and slowing down the aging process. The only other thing that can compare in terms of boosting HGH levels is high-intensity interval training which is covered later in this book!

✓ Lowers triglyceride levels by increasing fat burning.

✓ Helps suppress inflammation and fight free radical damage to lessen the risk of disease and chronic pain.

✓ Improve beneficial bacteria in your gut.

One thing I should point out is that Intermittent Fasting isn't easy for people to do, especially if you are used to eating several times a day. Doing this step by step in a logical manner to acclimate your body is a good way to go about things. This is also NOT an excuse to eat any food you want because you are only eating 6-10 hours of each day. If you eat a ton of crap food you will still look and feel like crap! No amount of fasting or hacks is going to help you with that! Now that you have all of these great reasons to give I.F a shot, here's a few ways how:

✓ **General Rules:** Eat foods that are good for you like lean meats, fruits, vegetables, protein powder, and healthy fats such as nuts, avocados, and olive/coconut oil. Definitely try to avoid refined carbs and sugar whenever possible.

✓ **Skip Breakfast:** This is quite possibly the easiest way to go about I.F. If you eat dinner around 7pm the night before, skip breakfast and make lunch (around 11am-12pm) your first meal of the day. It takes a few weeks for your body to start using fat as a preferential fuel source but once you do your sugar craving will go down tremendously!

✓ **Every other Day:** If fasting every day seems too much for you, try doing it every other day and eat as clean as possible every day of the week. Your body will still reap the benefits that day but it may not happen as quickly as a consistent fast would.

✓ **12 hour window:** If the idea of a 14-18 hour window makes you cringe, try to stop eating a few hours before bed and/or eat breakfast a few hours later to create a 12 hour window between meals. This will allow your body to digest and metabolize your food since it takes six to eight hours for your body to metabolize your glycogen stores (stored carbs). With a 12 hour fast, you can still reap some fat burning benefits.

✓ **Fasted Workouts:** As you learned, glycogen stores are burned up after 6-8 hours. If your last meal is at 6pm and you workout in the morning on an empty stomach at 8am, your body is more likely to utilize fat for energy rather than carbs. Working out during a fast has actually shown to increase fat burning and muscle oxidative capacity [28]. It may be a good idea to take some Branched Chain Amino Acids (BCAA's) (refer to hack #196) before, during, and after training to help with energy levels and repair muscle tissue. If you are lifting weights I recommend having a whey protein shake post fasted workouts. If you are just doing cardio, I recommend BCAA's and waiting to eat during the 6-10 hour "eating" window. The choice is yours.

If you don't feel well during Intermittent Fasting; STOP! This book is about making you healthier and although your body can go through transition phases during any dietary change causing you to feel fatigued, have cravings, etc; if after a couple of weeks you haven't become acclimated and haven't begun to feel better, stop and try something else.

49) GUT DIRTY?!

Your gut does more than tell you whether or not to 'go with it'. When everything works together, it's a beautiful thing, but when you start to have gut problems, boy can you feel it…and quite often smell it! Your gut's nervous system is a network of more than 100 million neurons that transmit information through electrical and chemical connections throughout your gastrointestinal (GI) tract. This system can operate the digestive system independently of your brain, deciding when to move food from the stomach to the small intestine, when to release hormones, when to drop waste, and even when to send food back out of your mouth when you are sick, yuck! Your gut truly has a mind of its own.

To make 'gut' decisions, your 'feel good' hormone serotonin, is in charge. In fact, 95% of your serotonin is made in your gut. The brain's serotonin helps create good feelings; the serotonin in the GI tract is its protection against bad bacteria and helps prevent inflammation. Signals are actually sent from the gut to the brain, not the other way around. When you are healthy you literally don't give these messages a second thought because your body is in equilibrium; but when you aren't feeling well, that's a different story. You can have bloating, pain, and irritability that can even emerge as anxiety and/or depression.

So to keep your gut happy, it's important to improve beneficial bacteria in your gut. Healthy gut bacteria, (which out numbers your cells ten to one), is one of the most important things you can do to improve your immune system to fight off illness. You will sleep better, have more energy, have increased mental clarity and improve your overall quality of life.

With all of this said how do we make sure our gut is healthy?

- ✓ **Exercise!** Exercise literally get things moving and can alleviate symptoms of Irritable Bowel Syndrome (IBS).

- ✓ **Chew your food!** Take your time to chew your food so that your digestive system doesn't have to work as hard. Digestion starts when you start chewing, not swallowing!

- ✓ **Take a probiotic.** The gut is host to tens of trillions of bacteria; 10 percent are "bad" (causing digestive distress) and 90 percent "good" (controlling the bad bacteria). *Probiotics* is just another word for "good bacteria." Ingested regularly, they'll help skew the ratio of bacteria in your gut in your favor. Look for bottles with 5 billion or more CFU (colony-forming units) and at least five strains of bacteria, with fun names to say like *Lactobacillus acidophilus;* trying saying that 5 times fast. Each person's gut is different, so if one probiotic isn't working, give another one a shot.

✓ **Peak-a-poop!** Gross! One of the easiest ways to check your gut health is to look into the toilet before you flush. Firm is good, hard could mean dehydration or constipation, and no shape means diarrhea. If your poop is skinny like a pen, red, or black you may want to see a doctor (unless you have eaten beets, as this can cause red feces).

✓ **Eat more fiber and drink more water.** If you suffer from constipation, try to consume 45-50 grams of fiber a day. Slowly increase your intake by 5 grams every couple of days until you become regular.

✓ **Cut back the alcohol and caffeine.** These are digestive stimulants and can cause you to have diarrhea.

✓ **Eat fermented foods.** Start using fermented vegetables as a side dish when you eat meat. Sauerkraut and Kimchi are a couple of examples. Kombucha tea is another example you can easily introduce as an evening habit. Also, if you can tolerate dairy, kefir is one of my favorites to mix with organic natural yogurt, dried fruit & nuts.

✓ **Eat Prebiotics:** Prebiotic foods are a type of plant fiber that feed the good bacteria already living in your digestive system. The more prebiotics and probiotics you eat the more efficiently the live bacteria will work. You can find prebiotics in foods such as asparagus, raw bananas, Jerusalem artichokes, leeks, oatmeal, red wine, onions, and legumes.

✓ **Avoid Common Triggers:** Avoid added sugars, refined grains, MSG, NSAIDs (such as ibuprofen or naproxen drugs), acid blockers, and alcohol (except red wine in moderate amounts).

If you try all of these and still have problems seek professional help from your healthcare provider as you may have a food allergy, a leaky gut, or other GI disorder.

50) CHEAT WITH CARB CYCLING!

You can't get lean without eating clean, but there are times when 'cheating' can actually assist in losing fat! Sweet, right?! This doesn't mean you can go crazy and say 'Joey told me to act like I'm a competitive eater!' What you can do is increase your carbohydrate intake (increasing your overall calorie intake) for a single day once or twice a week.

So here's why and how this works: Being on a restricted calorie diet can cause your levels of the critical hormone leptin to plummet. Leptin is in charge of keeping your hunger down and your metabolism up; so when its levels fall, you will essentially burn fewer calories. Carb cycling (overeating for your new calorie levels) jacks leptin levels back up, which keeps your metabolism elevated and your hunger suppressed. So when you return back to a lower calorie diet the next day, you will burn more calories while consuming less! Nice!

Here how to do it: Increase your carbs by 25-50% one or two days per week on non-consecutive days. Your body reaches equilibrium after 2-3 days and gets used to the lower calorie restriction; so increasing your calories one or two days a week provides a leptin and metabolism spike. Now if you keep your carbs clean by eating carbs like sweet potatoes, yams, wild rice, quinoa, beans, whole grains, red potatoes, and fruits, you will be on the right track! If you are resistance training and doing HIIT cardio (as you should be and find out why later in this book) it's best to complete your workouts on your carb cycling days to allow the carbs to fuel your workout and even further limit the possibility of fat gain. Now here it is…if you want to have that pizza, pasta, or cake you have been craving, this is the day to have your CHEAT meal; just don't make it a marathon cheat eating day!

51) KNOW WHAT TIME IT IS WITH NUTRITIONAL TIMING!

If we can properly time our macronutrients then we can utilize them to our advantage and prevent any sort of fat gain. One thing we can get control over is our carbs and when to eat them! As stated, I want you to avoid processed carbs when possible and get your complex carbs when they will benefit you the most. Here's a schedule of when you should eat your carbs:

- ✓ **Good Morning:** Eating your carbs in the morning is a good option as your body has essentially been fasting while you were asleep and glycogen levels (storage form of carbs) have been depleted. By eating carbs in the morning (with a protein of course), while insulin sensitivity is also higher, will allow you to replenish your lost glycogen. Your metabolic rate is higher in the morning allowing the carbs to literally fuel your day.

- ✓ **Better before exercise**: Before a high intensity workout. Have your carbs a few hours before your intense workout such as intervals, weights, resistance bands, or a sport. These carbs will be utilized to fuel your workout and refuel your body afterwards. This will limit any fat gain leaving you feel great!

- ✓ **Best after exercise:** The best time to consume carbs is after your workout when your body is primed to take in those nutrients and repair your body. Consuming the largest amount of your carbs post intense exercise is a great way to repair your body and possibly get your sweet fix in as well (learn more about this in hack #213)!

52) AVOID CHEMICALS!

Since 1940, over 75,000 synthetic chemicals have been created that often find their way into our food (even healthy foods) or in the food of the animals we eat. These chemicals have been shown to create an environment where we hold on to our fat and were coined "obesogens" first in 2006 by Professor Bruce Blumberg, a biology professor at the University of California, Irvine. The professor discovered that tin-based compounds known as organotins predisposed laboratory mice to gain weight [39]. The obesogens could be encouraging our body to hang on to fat by increasing their storage capacity, slowing down our metabolism (limiting amount of calories burned), have a negative effect on our gut biome, and trick our bodies into thinking we are still hungry.

So how do you avoid these chemicals?

- ✓ **Avoid Bisphenol-A (BPA):** We have all heard of BPA free but what is it?! BPA is a synthetic compound (found mostly in plastic food and drink containers). Studies show that BPA may increase fat-cell differentiation, disrupt pancreatic functioning, and cause insulin resistance, all of which can lead to obesity. So it's wise to stay away! Buy BPA-free bottles/food storage containers, avoid plastics marked with the #7 (in the recycling triangle) and avoid heating food/beverages in plastic containers. Be careful with canned foods, such as canned tomatoes (glass is a good option) and tuna fish. Canned tuna is one of the most BPA-laden foods on store shelves!

- ✓ **Eat Organic:** Triflumizole is a fungicide commonly used on many food crops, especially leafy greens, and has been linked to weight gain. Many of the chemicals used on our crops are endocrine disrupters; thus promoting fat storage and limiting our ability to build lean muscle [34]! Eat organic fruits and veggies or at the very least make sure these 14 types of foods, the 'dirty 14', are organic since they are known to have the highest levels of pesticides [35]:

✓ Apples	✓ Nectarines
✓ Celery	✓ Peaches
✓ Cucumbers	✓ Potatoes
✓ Cherry Tomatoes	✓ Snap Peas (Imported)
✓ Grapes	✓ Spinach
✓ Hot Peppers	✓ Strawberries
✓ Leafy Greens	✓ Sweet Bell Peppers

- ✓ **Avoid Emulsifiers:** These are chemicals that are added to processed foods to improve texture and prevent separation in foods like dips, salad dressing, and mayonnaise. These have been shown to contribute to weight gain and even cause gut issues and possible disease [34].

- ✓ **Stay away from processed foods** as the emulsifiers are hidden as 'polysorbates' and 'sorbitan monostearate' on food labels. As a result, you can take a healthy food, like a salad, and slather it in a not so healthy salad dressing full of emulsifiers! Eat whole foods and avoid these at all costs [34]!

- ✓ **Avoid Antibiotics and Hormones**! Our cattle and livestock are often pumped with antibiotics and hormones that can lower our immune function and cause us to gain weight (which is what they want the cattle to do). A study by the International Journal of Obesity found that the use of steroid hormones in conventional dairy farming and meat production could be a contributor to the obesity epidemic [34].

✓ **Choose lean cuts of meats** with little fat as the hormones are fat soluble. Choose antibiotic-free and hormone-free meats and dairy products (look for "organic," "free range" and "grass-fed" on the label).

Ways to detoxify your body:

✓ Your body wants to clean itself so you can facilitate the process by feeding it foods to help! Eat green veggies that are rich in chlorophyll like spinach and parsley and gelatinous plant foods like chia, aloe, sea weeds. Gels move through intestinal track and absorb and bind the bile salt released by the liver and gets rid of them.

✓ Parsley cleanses your blood supply and gives you fresh breath due to chlorophyll.

✓ Cilantro binds with heavy metals found in fish or dental fillings. Cilantro binds with the neurotoxin and removes it from your system.

Recap: Cleanse with greens, gelatinous foods, fresh filtered water and sunlight. Stay away from foods that have a longer shelf life than you!

53) CONTROL YOUR CRAVINGS!

Cravings for unhealthy foods are inevitable. I constantly hear 'I have to eat chocolate! If I don't, I end up caving in and ruining my diet!' Instead of caving all at once or having a 'cheat day', split your treats up into small bags. This way, when a craving comes and you need a fix of sweets, you can have the small portion that you have set aside; then carry on with your diet!

54) KNOW YOUR TRIGGERS!

As discussed in the previous hack there are ways to have small treats and remain healthy, but at the same time you have to know your triggers and what causes you to overeat, eat unhealthy foods, and derail your progress. I absolutely LOVE sweets and people often tell me to simply have one piece of cake, or one candy bar, to satisfy my cravings. Now this is sound advice, but I know myself; when I have sweets I literally eat until I feel sick! This is partially my fault since no one is force feeding me, but this is also caused by the chemical neuropeptide Y (NPY) response in the hypothalamus urging us to overeat uncontrollably [38]. Knowing this, I have to be honest with myself and realize that even eating one cookie will take me down a path of regret. Ask yourself, how I am going to feel when I eat this, and even more importantly, 'how am I going to feel after this?' If you are going to feel regret for overeating and derailing your health progress then simply DON'T eat it! Focusing on how you will feel after your 'FEED' will often make it much easier to say NO thanks! Now, if you do happen to eat that tray of brownies, don't use this as an excuse to give up on your health goals. YES, you messed up, IT HAPPENS, but quickly quit the pity party and get your health back on track!

55) PAY ATTENTION TO DISCOMFORTS!

Often, when starting on a new diet, we tend to dismiss certain pains or discomforts as 'our body getting used to the new foods'. However, you should be careful and get any abnormal sensitivity checked out because it may be that you have a dairy intolerance or lactose intolerance and an issue like this needs to be recognized.

56) MARK YOUR WATER!

This simple tip is probably one of the best I can give you. Next time you open a can of your favorite carbonated sugary drink; have a look at the contents and nutritional information. People often think that drinks cannot do any harm when on a diet but the opposite is actually true. Yes, that means even diet soda! There can be many hidden ingredients and calories in drinks so switching to water could be the best decision you make! A good way to make sure you are consuming enough water, especially in this busy world, is to use a marker or pen and draw marks on your reusable bottle; this will ensure you are drinking enough water by specific times of the day. Here's how: Get a large water bottle (glass or BPA free of course) and make marks (may be helpful to specify the time) on the bottle. For example, by 10am drink to the first mark you made, the next for mark is your goal by lunch, then by 3pm, etc. Before you know it drinking water throughout the day will be a habit!

57) YOUR PEE IS YOUR GUIDE!

How do you know if you are hydrated? Look at the color of your pee! If it is yellow/ dark yellow, it means that you need more fluids. If it is straw-colored, you are perfectly hydrated! If it is completely colorless, you could actually be drinking excess but I wouldn't worry about this one too much.

58) INFUSE YOUR WATER WITH FLAVOR!

So you're used to flavored beverages and the health benefits of plain old water aren't enough to get you to drink it. Well, simply infuse flavor into you water by adding fruit and herbs (like cucumber slices, blueberries, raspberries, citrus, basil and mint). Experiment with different flavor combinations that tickle your taste buds.

59) TRY LOCAL STORES!

Why not try the local meat supplier or the fruit and vegetable stand that you walk past every morning and night? The food at local shops is often fresher as they have a shorter farm to display journey compared to supermarkets. You may also find new foods that you haven't tried before!

60) GROW YOUR OWN FRUITS AND VEGETABLES!

This is extremely efficient but also, ultimately, REWARDING. Learn how to grow your own vegetables and you will save money from buying them in the long-run, plus you know EXACTLY where they came from! This way you don't have to worry about how they have been treated whilst growing. This can be great fun for the whole family!

61) STORE YOUR OWN FOODS!

Learn how to can food that you make using a simple mason jar. This way, they will keep for longer plus you don't have the worry of added nasties because you made it yourself!

62) FREEZE YOUR GREENS!

This is something my mother-in-law taught me. I love my green smoothies and often buy too many greens that they would go bad before I could use them. Freezing my greens solved that problem quick, how smart! Buy several bags of organic greens (if you can) and throw one or two of them in the freezer for your smoothies. The spinach, kale, Swiss chard, or whatever greens you have freeze very well and limit the need for added ice in your smoothies; making them cold, delicious, and YES, still nutritious!

63) JUST WOKE UP? EAT SOON!

If you like to eat breakfast try to eat within half hour of waking up as this can help to boost your metabolism and prepare your body and MIND for the day.

64) DON'T TRUST YOUR EYES!

One of the biggest problems that we face today is that we eat with our eyes. What do I mean by this? We buy into the bribes that are offered to us! Everything that we see is specifically designed to go against us. For example, in the supermarket, we are bombarded with temptations, from strategically placed displays to free sample day. Even when you are ready to checkout you can't escape it as we are surrounded with candy. This IS NOT a coincidence! Supermarkets know that we get hungry when shopping and that the bright packaging and yummy smells are going to draw us in! We have to remove this temptation from our lives; go to the supermarket when you know it will be quiet, concentrate on something else while you are in line like reading an article or thinking about your next healthy meal. You may want to shop online so you aren't tempted by treats at the grocery store and bring these 'little devils' into your home! If it isn't in your house, you can't eat it!

65) EAT ON A SMALLER PLATE!

We often use rather large dinner plates which makes nearly everything look small; causing us to fill our plates to the brim. Eating on a smaller plate also follows this thinking of our eyes deceiving us. The exact same meal will look bigger on a smaller plate! It is all about turning the odds in our favor [5]!

66) ALWAYS GO SHOPPING AFTER EATING!

This is the mistake that many of us make; we go shopping before eating so we are walking around hungry. When we are hungry, we tend to buy junk foods that we want to eat right now! If we go shopping on a full stomach, we are more likely to think ahead and less likely to buy unhealthy foods!

67) NO SNACKS IN THE BEDROOM!

Make sure that you DO NOT have any snacks in the bedroom as this can cause mindless eating. You tend to eat just because it is there!

68) HEALTHY SNACKS GALORE!

Make sure you have healthy snacks ready at every point in your day to satisfy any hunger that may strike! If we have healthy food ready, we will not be stopping into a fast-food outlet to grab a quick burger! Have snacks ready in your office, car, bag, etc.

69) WHEN IN ATHENS!

Do as the Greeks do! Make leftovers ON PURPOSE so that you have options available in the coming days. This can be particularly helpful if you know you have a busy few days ahead! My wife's family is Greek and every gathering from a few people to a few hundred people they will ALWAYS make too much food that NEVER goes to waste. Making extra portions of food can be stored and used for later in the week.

70) SECONDS?

You have just finished a beautiful Sunday roast dinner and you want more! But do you really? Sometimes it just takes a few minutes for our stomach to tell us that we are full so wait 10-20 minutes before you dive back in for seconds!

71) DO NOT TRUST THE MEDIA!

When it comes to food and drink, trust no one but yourself… and me of course. You have just seen a commercial promoting a new 'healthy' snack for kids! FANTASTIC! That will be a great addition to my child's lunchbox! STOP! Stop trusting commercials and things that you hear and take a look for yourself. You have to remember the advertising a company does for its product is to get YOU to buy it; so of course they will be throwing out all these 'healthy' claims left, right and center. Why not take a look at the packaging for yourself and decide whether it is healthy enough for your child? I'm talking to you, flavored milk companies!

72) REMEMBER BUSINESS PARTNERSHIPS!

Some companies form partnerships that seem contradictory to their core business model to promote each other's message no matter how crazy the claims seem. For example, the American Academy of Pediatric Dentistry agreed to a deal with Coca-Cola back in 2003, yes you read that right, dentists partnered with a soda company! As part of this agreement, Coca-Cola would distribute the academy's message about dental health. However, sugar has been proven to be the MAIN CAUSE of tooth decay! Not everything we see and hear can be trusted; I hate to say it but money seems to be the driving force for most companies while our health is a VERY low priority!

'Food for Life' Hacks

73) WAKE UP and take a SHOT!

No, not that kind of shot! My morning elixir shot! Every morning when you wake up, have a glass of warm water with the juice from one lemon, 2 tablespoons of Organic Apple Cider Vinegar (ACV), a few dashes of cayenne pepper (optional), and a teaspoon of cinnamon. Lemon juice is well known for aiding digestion as well as cleansing the system. ACV will help with digestion, reduce blood sugar levels, and has also been shown to reduce the blood sugar spike of a high carb meal by 19-34%; leading to less fat gain! Try 2 tablespoons of ACV before any high carb/sugary meal! Cayenne pepper boasts helpful detoxification properties and will complement the lemon juice well, but is not to everyone's taste. The cinnamon in the shot provides increased health benefits like decreased inflammation, blood sugar regulation, and antioxidants.

74) CAULIFLOWER RICE!

Traditional white rice and even brown rice can be EXTREMELY calorific which can be a huge problem when planning meals. Shredding a cauliflower can be a great alternative to significantly lowering the amount of calories sitting on your plate. One cup of cauliflower has 27 calories, 5 grams of carbs, 2.7 grams of fiber and 2 grams of protein! One cup of white rice has 205 calories, 44 grams of carbs, NO FIBER, and 4 grams of protein (brown rice is better in that it has the fiber still intact)! If you find the taste rather bland, add some of your favorite herbs or spices to give it a delicious kick!

75) LETTUCE BE MY BREAD!

Bread for sandwiches as well as buns for burgers can be a huge hit on your daily calorie intake; so why not try switching it out for something new? Lettuce can be a great replacement! Using lettuce as a base for your sandwich fillings or burgers can be EXTREMELY satisfying and refreshing! Lettuce is really low in calories and pretty much a freebie any time of the day…go ahead and try to gain weight eating greens, I dare you!

76) GET YOUR CALCIUM!

Calcium has been shown in numerous studies to build muscle and enhance fat loss, especially around the old spare tire! This could be due to the hormone calcitrol, which promotes fat gain and limits fat burning. Calcitrol is suppressed when adequate calcium is consumed in the diet. Calcium has also been shown to decrease the amount of dietary fat absorbed by your intestines, and some studies even suggest it can curb your appetite.

Dairy products are known to be high in calcium, like low-fat cottage cheese and Greek yogurt, but you don't need to eat dairy to get your calcium (MIND BLOWN!) Other sources include: sunflower seeds (which are also high in mono-unsaturated/polyunsaturated fats), spinach, soybeans, kale, figs (also high in fiber and potassium), almonds (and almond milk), flaxseeds, and even oranges! Try to eat foods high in calcium three times a day; and if you don't get enough consider supplementing with a vitamin.

77) 'NO' TO UNHEALTHY OILS!

Oils are required in a lot of cooking but that doesn't mean they have to be bad for you. Try replacing unhealthy oils and fats with coconut oil. Coconut oil helps to burn fat and is also more filling so it can reduce the need for snacking later. Coconut oil can also help with brain health, prevent heart disease and high blood pressure, reduces inflammation, possible cancer prevention, boosts your immune system, improves energy, and improves digestion to name a few. It's also great for a moisturizer and makes you smell like a tropical drink, yum! Other healthy oils include but not limited to: avocado oil, olive oil, almond oil, grapeseed, and walnut oil.

78) NATURAL SWEETENERS!

Refined sugars can be detrimental to your health as they contribute to the amount of fat stored in your body. Replacing these with natural sweeteners such as stevia or honey removes this problem as you will be taking in fewer calories as well as enjoying a lower blood sugar count!

79) SWAP OUT REGULAR FLOUR!

Refined bleached flour can do extreme harm to your body and spike your blood sugar leading to a host of potential issues; but that doesn't mean you still can't bake. Just opt for one of these better alternatives:

- ✓ **Coconut flour**- made from the coconut meat after most its fat has been extracted to produce coconut oil. Coconut flour is low carb, rich in fiber, and is gluten free! You will need to modify your recipes to add more liquid as the fiber absorbs a lot of water. A 1/4 cup of coconut flour contains 60 calories, 2.5 g of fat, 6 g of protein, 19 g of carbohydrates and 12 g of fiber, awesome! If you look at the net carbs of coconut flour (the total carbs minus the fiber content), the net carbs are the carbs that can raise your blood sugar levels. Coconut flour has a net carb content of 7 g per 1/4-cup serving. Whereas the same serving of all-purpose wheat flour contains 24 g of carbs, 0.8 g of fiber, or 23.2 g of net carbs; and 1/4 cup of whole-wheat flour has 22 g of carbs and 3.2 g of fiber, or 18.8 g of net carbs. Simply by switching to coconut flour you are saving between 11-15g of net carbs!

- ✓ **Almond meal** - Another low carb flour that won't cause blood sugar levels to spike drastically is almond meal. You can make your own by grinding almonds until you get a fine flour-like consistency. Don't grind for too long or you will get almond butter; although homemade almond butter is delicious! You can also buy almond meal at many grocery stores. You can use almond meal to make any of your favorite recipes; just be aware that since it is gluten free it doesn't rise as much. Each 1/4 cup of almond meal contains 5.2 g of carbohydrates and 2.9 g of fiber, which leaves only 2.3 g of net carbs.

✓ **Walnut meal** – Walnuts can be ground into flour or be purchased in a grocery store as well. Walnuts are an excellent choice as they are high in alpha-linolenic acid, a type of omega-3 fatty acid that is good for your heart health. Each 1/4 cup of ground walnuts provides 2.7 g of carbs and 1.3 g of fiber, which corresponds to 1.4 g of net carbs. You can also use macadamia nuts, hazelnuts or pistachios. Now just because you replaced a high carb flour with a low carb one doesn't mean you should add a bunch of other unhealthy ingredients into your food (like extra sugar). It's the little things that will make a BIG difference!

80) VEGGIE NOODLES!

Normal grain-based noodles are pretty calorific so why not switch to a more natural based noodle. Why not try zucchini or butternut squash as your noodle replacement? They will be far healthier and you can have some fun finding your favorite variation! You can even buy an inexpensive gadget that shreds veggies in long noodle-like strands!

81) PROTEIN POWDER!

I often get asked 'How do I get more protein? It's impossible to get enough when eating healthy!' Actually it's easy. One great way of increasing your protein intake is to use protein powder when cooking. It can be used to replace some of the required flour, for example, when cooking pancakes; make protein pancakes instead…yummy (see hack below)!

82) PROTEIN PANCAKES!

Here, we have a delicious protein cinnamon pancake for you to try for breakfast!

Give this **Protein Pancake** recipe a shot:

INGREDIENTS:

- ✓ 1/4 cup egg whites
- ✓ 1 banana
- ✓ 1 serving of protein powder
- ✓ 1 tsp ground cinnamon
- ✓ 1/4 cup oats
- ✓ 1/4 unsweetened milk (almond, cashew, coconut, or milk), may have to add more (or less)

depending on consistency and amount of protein powder.

- ✓ 1 tbsp. ground flax seed (great source of protein, fiber, Omega-3 fats, and makes your skin, hair, and nails strong and healthy!)

DIRECTIONS:

1. Mash your RIPE banana, add all of the ingredients and mix in a bowl. Use a non-stick pan on medium heat with cooking spray or coconut oil. Place some of the batter on to the pan and wait for it to bubble (about 30 seconds to a minute). Flip over for no more than 30 seconds and remove from pan. Continue the process with the rest of the batter. This should make 4-8 pancakes depending on size. Top with fresh fruit, Greek yogurt, or organic nut butter and enjoy! These also go well on the run as a snack or left in the fridge for later eating pleasure.

NUTRITION INFO (varies based on protein powder) About 250 calories, 5.5g fat, 18g carbs, and 31.8g of protein!

83) BE SMOOTHIE IN ADVANCE!

If you tend to get a craving for something sweet at a similar time every day, be pre-pared and use it to your advantage. Pre-chop some fruit (or use frozen) along with other HEALTHY ingredients, so that as soon as the craving hits, all you have to do is put it all into a blender and be ready in no time flat! EASY PEASY! If you don't get enough (like most of us) add some spinach or kale in a blender with fruit to get all of the green goodness for your body! If you are one of 'those people' who won't eat anything green place the drink in a colored container so you don't see it...or close your eyes while chugging away! Another great option is to add some protein powder and/or nut butter for some extra protein and healthy fats to keep you full! Up until a few years ago I wouldn't eat ANYTHING green unless it was candy, seriously! I started by adding greens to my protein smoothies and now I crave vegetables, salads, and healthy food...my mother doesn't know where her little "sugarholic" boy went!

84) PLATE YOUR COLD GREENS!

You are more likely to eat less if cold raw greens are on your plate. WHY? Because cold raw greens like spinach or lettuce generally take up more room on the plate and also require more chewing so you feel as though you are eating more! Generally the darker the better and more nutritionally dense (try spinach, kale, Swiss chard, etc.).

85) EAT DARK POULTRY!

For a long time, the theory has been that the lighter parts of a chicken, like the breast for example, have far less calories than the darker parts, such as the thighs. It is true that there are fewer calories, but according to recent tests, it is only about 10 calories per pound. The chicken breast is often drier so we tend to throw on condiments to compensate which actually makes the whole choice worthless. The thigh is normally moist and contains more flavors thus removing the need for added condiments and saving calories!

86) INCREDIBLE EDIBLE EGG!

'I will have an egg white omelet please!' Less calories? Yes. Healthier? Well, there is room for improvement. See the YOLK contains many vital nutrients; therefore the entire egg should be eaten. Egg yolks came under fire in the 20th century when a study on rabbits was conducted. Rabbits were fed PURE cholesterol and their arteries became clogged with plaque. It was concluded that anything with cholesterol and fat promoted heart disease. This study doesn't hold much validity, since eggs are not naturally in a rabbit's diet! Even *Time Magazine reversed the argument* it made in a 1984 cover story claiming eggs and other high-fat foods were dangerous, and even encouraged readers to eat butter over margarine, mmm butter!

Here's the hard boiled truth about yolks:

Whole eggs are a nearly perfect food, with almost every essential vitamin and mineral our bodies need to function. It is one of the few natural food sources of vitamin D and contains 7 grams of high-quality protein to fuel your muscles. Whole eggs are also full of omega-3 fatty acids and deliver many of the B vitamins (for energy) and nutrients B6, B12, riboflavin, folate, and choline. Eggs are believed to help reduce heart disease. They have L-arginine (an amino acid) which is critical to the body's production of protein and the release of growth hormone to help with weight loss and metabolism. Another amino acid found in eggs, leucine, also helps the body produce growth hormone as well as regulate blood sugar levels leading to lower incidence of fat storage. The yolk itself contains *most* of these vitamins and minerals, plus half of its protein.

When you eat only the egg whites, you're missing out on all of these nutritional benefits and are getting only 3.5 grams, or half, of the protein. Be sure to opt for cage-free or free range organic eggs, as chickens cooped up in a cage tend to produce eggs with less nutritional value. Here's the low down: as long as you control your calories, egg yolks are a MUST in your diet, even with their fat content. If you are watching your calories I would rather you cut something else out of your diet besides the egg yolks; even if you have to order an omelet with one or two yolks and the rest whites. Now if you are eating the yolks with pancakes, sausage, bacon, and dessert, then all of the eggs in the world won't save you! Now that's no YOLK, haha!

87) SIDE SAUCE!

This rule mainly applies when eating in a restaurant or around other people but have your sauces on the side! That way YOU are in control of how much goes on and not the chef! Also, you may never really know what ingredients are sauces like barbeque sauce, which often contains corn syrup and other sweeteners.

88) DON'T RUIN THE SALAD!

So you have decided to eat a salad, good choice, but then it suddenly gets ruined with a thick creamy UNHEALTHY calorific fatty salad dressing! Why not try using vinaigrette instead and save yourself the heartbreak when you step onto the scale.

89) NO MORE MILK!

Alternatives to fatty cow's milk, like **unsweetened** almond, cashew, and coconut milk can contain half the amount of calories than even SKIMMED milk. While 2% (skim milk contains added sugar), is a better option than full-fat, there are still better options out there (especially if you are a coffee addict). Just remember, when choosing milk substitutes go for unsweetened, not vanilla, not chocolate, not original, but unsweetened...got it?

90) POWDERED PEANUT BUTTER!

This can offer four times LESS calories than the same amount of the real thing but still gives you the great peanut taste! It is designed to be made with water or can even be added to your smoothies. Here's what I do with it; I take 2 tablespoons of powdered peanut butter (about 45 calories as opposed to almost 200 for regular peanut butter), add some cinnamon, a little cashew milk or water, stir it up and enjoy on an apple or carrots, yum! You just saved yourself a couple hundred calories! If peanuts aren't your thing, you can find a variety of powdered nut butters.

91) YOU DON'T WHITE BREAD?

You should really try to avoid white bread at all costs. There are better alternatives so you shouldn't find a need for white bread. For example, whole grain bread often has a similar amount of calories but it fills you up more so you can keep going for longer. If you aren't willing to kick the white bread completely use one piece of whole grain bread and one piece of white bread. As a general rule, the darker the better…unless its chocolate flavored of course!

92) GREEK YOGURT for MAYO!

Greek yogurt is thought to contain 10 TIMES more protein than mayonnaise! So next time you get the mayo out of the fridge remember that Greek yogurt is a much better alternative.

93) PLAIN YOGURT!

Flavored yogurt can contain up to 15 grams more sugar than plain; 15 GRAMS! Knowing this, it seems silly to go for anything else other than plain! Add fruit, cinnamon, mixed nuts, seeds, or a nut butter to add flavor without the extra refined sugar!

94) YOGURT LIQUID!

Often when you lift the lid off of a yogurt you see a layer of liquid sitting on top. Your instinct may be to drain it, but DON'T throw it away. This liquid actually contains valuable whey protein. So mix it in and don't let it put you off. Think of the long-term benefits!

95) FRUIT IN YOUR BREAKFAST!

This can sweeten the start to your day as well as add texture. Try adding a nice ripe, chopped apple to your oatmeal, yogurt or healthy breakfast.

96) AVOCADO ON TOAST

Ever notice how soft ripe avocado is? Use this to your advantage and spread it over a slice of toast (whole grain bread, of course!) to start your day with a kick! Avocado can also be used as a replacement for mayo in tuna (get the white tuna in water), add some creaminess to tacos instead of cheese, and even add it to your smoothies for great texture, healthy fats, and much needed fiber!

97) SAY 'HEALTHY GRILLED CHEESE!'

So you have decided you want a grilled cheese? On its own, this isn't the healthiest option so you have to improvise. Why not use whole grain bread, or make a cauliflower crust, and add sliced tomatoes, avocado or leafy greens?

98) SOUP TOO BORING?

Add some vegetables to your plain soup! You may have picked up a can of soup because it is a quick option. You may say 'I don't have time to chop up veggies' and you don't have to if you use canned or frozen vegetables. Side note: if you are grabbing a premade can of soup go for one with the least sodium, you can always add salt if you need more but you can't ever take away!

99) SMOOTHIES FOR BREAKFAST!

Try replacing your cereal with a smoothie! Smoothies are a fantastic way to get vital vitamins and fill your body with goodness for the day ahead. Use your favorite fruits and try different combinations! Add some protein powder if you like as well; vanilla or chocolate all natural/organic protein powder goes very well!

100) COFFEE!

Avoid the calorific, high sugar coffees that are on sale nowadays and stick to plain black coffee which is just less than 5 calories. Sipping on coffee or green tea throughout the day will keep your energy levels high and reduce the risk of you crashing when you get home from work (meaning that you will be ready for a workout!). If you need some flavor add cinnamon, coconut oil, or an unsweetened milk alternative (cashew, flax, coconut, or hemp milk are great options).

101) ORDERLY MEALS!

A classic mistake when eating our meals is to fill ourselves up on food that isn't going to give us the nutrients we need! Try to eat the protein and greens on your plate first as they are more rewarding as well as filling. You can then finish the meal off if you are truly hungry. Eating protein and greens first has been shown to limit the blood sugar spike of your food as opposed to eating the carbs first; so tell those French fries to wait until you enjoy your salad. Who knows, you may not eat them all!

102) YOUR CARBS SHOULD NEVER BE LONELY!

NEVER eat refined carbs, or as some people use the term 'impact carbs' by themselves. Impact carbs tend to spike blood sugar (raise insulin) more than other foods which create a fat storing environment inside our body. In fact, it's nearly impossible to burn fat in the presence of high insulin. Combine your impact carbs with some type of lean protein. Avoid breads (white), cookies, cakes, pies, and any sweets!

103) SWAP BREAD CRUMBS WITH GLUTEN FREE OATS!

Recipe calls for bread crumbs? Grind up some gluten free oats and use those instead for a more nutritious lower calorie option!

104) HALF POTATO, HALF CAULIFLOWER!

The next time you are making mashed potatoes for your meal, swap half of the potato for cauliflower. This will lessen the amount of carbs and sugars you are consuming as well as add fiber to make you full. Best of all, it still tastes delicious!

105) AN APPLE A DAY!

Ever wonder how you can pre-slice an apple ahead of time without it turning brown by snack time? Place slices in a baggie or container and squeeze some lemon juice on top. Seal and shake so your apples will retain their color! Plus the lemon juice adds a bit of tartness that goes great with the sweet apple flavor. Apples also contain antioxidants called polyphenols that boost strength, endurance, and aid in fat loss, especially around the midsection! Apples are a great option at any point during the day and for a little pre-workout snack!

106) SNACK HEALTHY!

Snacking can often be the downfall of a diet, people say 'well, I eat all three of my meals are healthy and I have cut out sweets, chocolate, and soda, but I'm still not losing weight!' The most common reason for this is the snacks that we take IN BETWEEN meals. Sometimes you don't even realize how much you snack over the course of a day because you almost do it subconsciously. Try raw fruits and vegetables, hard boiled eggs, as well as nuts and seeds to ensure you are making the most of your snacks! Be sure to only have one or two servings and not 10! Snacks are essentially foods to get us through to the next meal; so let's go back to basics and snack how we should!

107) DON'T OVERLOAD ON CARBS!

Some carbohydrates make good additions for a healthy meal like sweet potatoes, quinoa, brown rice, couscous, barley, whole grains, and more. But overloading on carbs will have a negative effect. You still need to think about what you are eating to ensure you are consuming all the important nutrients.

108) QUINOA FOR RICE!

Quinoa has THREE TIMES as much fiber and TWICE as much protein as regular rice! Quinoa is great because it will absorb the flavor of the sauce. Try it in soup, chili, or even as a swap to pasta.

109) MUSTARD!

If you are used to using calorific and fatty sauces to garnish your plate, try using mustard as a replacement. It contains no sugar or saturated fat! Mustard also has anti-inflammatory properties, can help you lose weight with complex B vitamins like folate, niacin, thiamine, and riboflavin which can speed up your metabolism. Mustard has also been shown to lower cholesterol, slow down aging from antioxidants, and stimulates hair growth from beta carotene which gets converted into vitamin A.

110) TEA IS YOUR FRIEND!

This one particularly applies to those who drink a lot of sugary drinks; try drinking tea instead. Tea contains no sugar (unless you add it in, of course) compared to a soda which can contain up to 8 TEASPOONS. Another benefit of tea is the antioxidants that it packs which can have a fantastic impact on your body! Try Green tea for amazing antioxidant properties and metabolic boost, black tea for a caffeine fix, and even roasted dandelion tea to reduce bloat and excess water weight (see hack #123).

111) NUTTY SALAD!

Salad is quite clearly a good option as a meal, but often croutons are included. If you swap these for almonds, you will reap the benefits. Almonds contain FAR MORE fiber and protein and FAR LESS carbohydrates. Other great options are pistachios, cashews, walnuts, or any other nut for some crunch.

112) POPCORN!

A standard lunch contains a packet of potato chips but these are EXTREMELY damaging to your diet. Replacing them with air popped popcorn (without butter) would ensure that you consume 35 less calories per ounce as well as NINE TIMES less saturated fat!

113) STEVIA!

Stevia is a 100% natural sugar-replacement that has zero CALORIES, CARBS OR SUGAR, and doesn't spike your blood sugar! A morning cup of tea with stevia will do your body wonders!

114) CACAO NIBS!

This can be a great replacement for chocolate chips as they contain no sugar and over FIVE TIMES more fiber!

115) ROMAINE LETTUCE!

Iceberg lettuce is obviously a great, healthy choice to keep calories low but you can get EVEN BETTER in the nutrient department! One head of romaine lettuce contains about FOUR TIMES more vitamin A than carrots as well as 535% of your RDA of vitamin K; so it is something to consider when planning next week's salads. Added Bonus: Remember the importance of sleep? Romaine lettuce contains lactucarium (the white fluid you see when you break the leaves) which has sleep inducing properties. So feel free to snack on it before bed.

116) CHIA SEEDS!

After hearing the benefits of using chia seeds, you will have no reason not to use them. I hope you are ready. Chia seeds are packed with fiber, protein, and are low sodium! Chia seeds are also known to take toxins out of our bodies and excrete them in our waste because they can absorb 9 times their own volume. Use Chia seeds in your salads, yogurt, oatmeal, shakes, or any other meal, just watch your teeth, they have a sneaky way of getting in between them; so have your toothpick ready.

117) SALT ALTERNATIVES!

Himalayan Pink Salt can be used as a great alternative to your regular table salt as it contains minerals and trace elements in their natural, unprocessed form.

118) COCONUT WATER!

There have been many debates on what to drink during, but especially after exercising. Recently, the rise of sports drinks has been astronomical but there is a healthier alternative. Recent studies have shown that COCONUT WATER can be highly beneficial during, before, and after exercise; as it contains over 16 times the amount of potassium, but less than half of the sugars compared to a sports drink! There is NO need to have a fancy sports drink loaded with sugar anymore. I know, I know, the marketing is so good!

119) CINNAMON!

Cinnamon is AMAZING for lowering the glycemic index of food! It is also known to help with other health problems like diabetes (as it lowers blood sugar), the common cold and even erectile dysfunction! Use cinnamon anytime you want some sweetness and to lower the glycemic index (sugar spike) in the foods you are eating.

120) CONTROL SODIUM!

There is no doubt about it, sodium is bad for us! It makes our bodies hold onto A LOT of water and we bloat as a result. To reduce the effect of this, we should try to keep our sodium intake between (or below) 1500-2300mg per day (that's under 1 teaspoon of salt which has 2,352mg). The foods with the highest levels of sodium include, but not limited to, table salt, cheese and sauces/dressings. When available, opt for the low sodium version.

121) GRAPEFRUIT BEFORE A BAD MEAL!

Eating some grapefruit or drinking a glass of fresh squeezed grapefruit juice before a unhealthy meal can be EXTREMELY helpful as it will lower the blood sugar spike of the food you are about to consume; making it less likely to be stored as fat! According to a study out of Scripps Clinic in San Diego, California, found that people eating half a grapefruit or eight ounces of fresh squeezed grapefruit juice three times a day lost on average four pounds in 12 weeks; probably due to the insulin lowering effects and metabolic boosting properties! Besides having half of a grapefruit before a bad meal try adding half to your breakfast and one half at lunch! Before adding grapefruit to your diet make sure it does not interfere with any medication you are currently taking.

122) SUPERFRUITS TO THE RESCUE!

Guava is a popular fruit at the moment because of its levels of vitamin C; helping to make your skin look young and wrinkle free. It is recommended to have at least five portions of fruit a day, so make most of them SUPER with these great options; Pichuberries and the South African Maqui berry, both of which are high in anti-oxidants, the nervous system protecting Camu Camu berry from the Amazon, the immune boosting Goji berry that also promotes healthy levels of Human Growth Hormone (HGH), and the fruit known to clear up the sinuses the Asian fruit Red Jujube date.

123) DANDELION ROOT TEA!

Drink this to reduce the amount of water you hold! Increased water weight makes you feel bloated and uncomfortable! Dandelion tea can help to remove this as it acts as a diuretic and makes you urinate more! However, because of its diuretic properties it is best to avoid if you are pregnant.

124) NO CHEWING – ONE DAY A WEEK!

This can be great to give your digestive system a break! Think of how hard your digestive system is working 24/7; it never gets a rest! When you have finished your meal, its work has only just begun! Try having a day where you consume only smoothies, shakes, or fruit and veggie juices!

125) SNACK ON FAT!

'Seems like a contradiction to me. One minute you are saying eat less, now eat more?' Snacking on healthy fats, like a handful of almonds, can actually be useful as they fill us up and we are then likely to consume fewer calories in the day because we aren't as hungry! Healthy fats are great to have before going out to dinner because they will make you feel full and less likely to eat a lot of bad food. Other great options are hard boiled eggs, shredded unsweetened coconut, and avocados (see below).

126) ALL ABOUT AVOCADOS!

Avocados have an unjust reputation of being 'high in fat', and that is true, but most of this 'fat' is monounsaturated which is healthy for the heart. Avocados are known to lower cholesterol and the US government has recently suggested that we eat more, just in moderation! Oddly enough, I actually agree with the government on this one.

127) LET'S GO NUTS!

Walnuts, pistachios and almonds all contribute to our diet more than we could imagine! Walnuts contain a natural omega-3 fatty acid, pistachios have qualities that bring benefits to our eye health, and almonds are rich in vitamin E. Research suggests that nut eaters are less likely to develop Type 2 diabetes and have a reduced risk of heart disease. Those benefits alone should be enough to make us all go nuts! As well as these, Brazil nuts also carry some great health benefits! Brazil nuts are high in selenium which can significantly reduce our chances of getting skin cancer.

128) BATCHES OF SOUP!

Making soup in batches is a GREAT idea! You know that it is flavorful because YOU made it and it can be kept and stored for the days ahead! Separate the batch into containers and you have your lunch for the next couple of days (you can even place them in the freezer to have when you need)! Soup is also a good choice if you are on the go as it is filling and can reduce hunger when you are out and about!

129) DAILY DESSERTS?

Do we need a dessert after every single meal or has it become a habitual ritual embedded in our brains? Try having a dessert every other day after one meal until you are able remove them completely. Once you stop consuming desserts on a daily basis, you will wonder why you had them every day! If you do miss eating 'something' after dinner, replace it with a healthy dessert like a fruit salad or a square of dark chocolate (at least 75% cacao to reap the benefits). Getting healthy is all about breaking bad habits and replacing them with good ones.

130) GINGER TEA!

Ginger is fantastic at helping digestion so be sure to drink some warm ginger tea before and after dinner! Ginger contains gingerol along with other oils that will prevent bloating and aid digestion! It can also be helpful to sip the drink during dinner; a much better option than fizzy drinks which have the opposite effect!

131) FLAX SEEDS!

Flax seeds can be great to add into a shake or salad as they help to lower cholesterol levels as well as help to control blood sugar levels! One serving (two tablespoons) can contain a healthy amount of fiber as well as DOUBLE the recommended amount of alpha-linolenic acid (which is a heart-healthy omega-3 fatty acid)!

132) NOTHING SOUR ABOUT VINAIGRETTE!

Make a batch of vinaigrette and keep it in the fridge for use on salads along with anything else you want to try it on! If homemade, vinaigrettes are a much healthier option than creamy dressings. A simple vinaigrette consists of; ¾ cup of healthy oil mixed in with ¼ cup of vinegar (or lime juice) along with a bit of salt! You can then play around with your favorite herbs and seasonings until it tastes perfect!

133) CHIPOTLE KICK!

It is often assumed that eating healthy is 'bland' and boring,' however this couldn't be further from the truth; you just have to find the flavors! A good way of adding a kick to your meal is to mix up a can of chipotle chilies in a blender into a paste; this can then be used to complement many dishes adding a delicious smoky kick! You can also make up a batch and store it in the fridge!

134) EAT SKIN!

'Huh?' is probably the most common response to this tip. Eating the skin of a kiwi has many benefits! You lose nearly 15% of all the nutrients that a kiwi holds when you peel it, that's a significant amount that can be beneficial to your health just thrown in the garbage! The skin also delivers extra fiber; but be sure to give it a good wash!

Other Foods you should eat with the skin:

- ✓ Apples: for their fiber, vitamin C, and vitamin A (lose about 1/3 of these nutrients without the skin).

- ✓ Potatoes: the skin contains iron, calcium, potassium, magnesium, and vitamins B6 and C.

- ✓ Peel of an Orange: twice the Vitamin C as the inside, contains riboflavin, B6, calcium, magnesium, potassium, and cancer fighting inflammatory properties (citrus also boosts iron absorption).

- ✓ Cucumbers: the skin contains most of the antioxidants, fiber, vitamin K, and potassium.

- ✓ Eggplant: the skin contains an antioxidant called nasunin which helps protect against cancer.

- ✓ Mango: the skin contains resveratrol, which helps burn fat and inhibits production of fat cells, nice!

✓ Watermelon: the rind has the most citrulline which is an amino acid that is converted into arginine which is essential for the heart, immune system, and circulatory system.

135) SUNBATHE LIKE A MUSHROOM!

Humans are like mushrooms in that we both produce vitamin D when exposed to the sun! In fact, just FIVE MINUTES in the sun and the vitamin D levels in mushrooms can be significantly boosted (to the point where they provide over 800% of our recommended daily allowance so eat up). Just make sure to put your sunscreen on after your 5 minutes of sunlight; we want Vitamin D, not skin cancer.

136) ARE YOUR PEARS RIPE?

Many of us check the body of the pear to see if it is ready to eat when we should actually be checking the neck. Pears generally ripen from the inside out so by the time the body feels 'soft', it is often too late! Pears are a good source of fiber, potassium, and Vitamin B2, C, E.

137) LEMON PLEASE!

Lemon juice is full of antioxidants so you CANNOT go wrong from adding some to your tea or water to give it a refreshing flavor. Reap the many benefits including:

✓ The reduction of inflammation: lemon may taste acidic but it actually helps alkalize the body and reduce inflammation by reducing uric acid in your joints.

✓ Aids in digestion by loosening toxins in your digestive tract and helps to relieve symptoms of indigestion such as heartburn, burping, and bloating (guys drink this before a hot date; no farts on the first date…maybe the second!).

✓ Lemons contain pectin fiber, which assists in fighting hunger cravings.

✓ Naturally cleanses your system by flushing out toxins by enhancing enzyme function and stimulating your liver. In fact, lots of bodybuilders and models will drink lemon water for days before a photoshoot because they feel that it makes their skin tighter and less bloated, I've done this and I agree!

✓ Lemons also help keep your skin blemish and possibly wrinkle free by their antioxidant power (no Botox!).

✓ Lemons also provide an excellent source of vitamin C to boost your immune system when you are stressed, provide potassium for heart health, and can even help viral infections, wow, that's a lot!

So how much do you use? It's all a matter of preference, usually a half of a lemon squeezed into a glass of water is good, but if you like the taste of lemon go nuts and squeeze the entire thing!

138) EAT PROTEIN LATE!

'What?!' But I thought eating late at night wasn't a good thing?!' Yes, in general you don't want to have a massive meal before you get to bed as your body will more likely store the excess calories as fat as opposed to utilizing it as energy. If you want to eat something late at night, a lean protein with greens and/or a healthy fat is an excellent option. Eating protein before bedtime means that the amino acids from your meal will be utilized as fuel for your muscles and your brain while you sleep. A great option would be to pair a greens salad with a chicken breast and nuts, a turkey lettuce wrap with avocado, or plain Greek yogurt or low fat cottage cheese (sprinkled with walnuts). Think of it as a 'protein IV' as you sleep. *Note if you want to add muscle try casein protein shake at night, this is a slower absorbing protein and provides your muscles with a constant supply of protein throughout the night.

139) MAKE YOUR NUTS COLD!

BRRR! If walnuts are kept in temperatures that are too warm, their oils can become rancid and the healthy snack can turn into a slightly less healthy option. Keeping them in a fridge or freezer will slow this process down and help maintain their crunch!

140) YOGURT TO FIX BAD BREATH!

Yogurt is known to be helpful in eliminating bad breath and keeping the bad bacteria that settle in your mouth! Try incorporating 6 ounces of Greek yogurt a day; as the good bacteria found in the yogurt overpower the bad bacteria, keeping bad breath at bay!

141) EASE THAT MIGRAINE!

Low magnesium levels are to blame for a bad migraine so the solution to this is simple – eat foods high in magnesium! Pumpkin seeds can be great for this as one cup contains just over 40% of our daily allowance. Other foods include cashews, almonds, peas, broccoli, oatmeal, flaxseed, and bananas.

142) OILY PEANUT BUTTER!

We have discovered that the liquid on top of yogurt is a big YES, however, the liquid you get on top of peanut butter is a big NO! This is oil and can be extremely damaging to our diet; for each tablespoon of oil you remove, you remove OVER 110 CALORIES as well as 14 GRAMS OF FAT! These are hidden nasties that you may not have even thought about before but can add up quickly!

143) WATER = LESS CONSTIPATION!

This is a great tip if you get constipated FREQUENTLY and it is a habit we should all practice; DRINK MORE WATER! Your body removes water as the stool passes through your intestines so keeping hydrated can be vital for ensuring enough water remains to allow the stool to pass easily!

144) FIBER UP AND POOP IT OUT!

Have you ever wondered why doctors tell us to eat more fiber when it comes to constipation? Fiber in your stool helps attract more water and therefore help keep the stool soft! However, if you consume too much fiber and not enough water, the stool will become hard once again! As a result of this, the recommended daily intake of fiber stands at around 25-30 grams! Make sure to get plenty of soluble and insoluble fiber. The soluble will make you feel full from your food and the insoluble will get thing moving through you, literally! If you don't get enough fiber from your diet try adding a fiber supplement (see below for one).

145) TAKE YOUR PSYLLIUM LIKE GRANDPA!

Psyllium brings A LOT of health benefits to our diet however, not many people are completely aware of them. Psyllium is a fiber that comes from a shrub-like herb and is known as a fantastic combative option to high cholesterol as well as reducing the risk of cancer, high blood pressure, diabetes, heart disease, diverticulosis and more. It also helps to improve irritable bowel, gas, diarrhea and constipation. 'Where can I get this magical fiber?' you may ask. Psyllium can often be found as the main ingredient in a lot of high-fiber cereals (take a look at the ingredients next time you shop, you will be surprised). You can also find it in ice cream! Believe it or not, a single serving of ice cream can actually have MORE FIBER than a slice of whole grain bread. The call for healthier desserts in recent times have meant that manufacturers are using psyllium fiber as a thickening agent to compensate for the high levels of fat and cholesterol in such a treat. This doesn't mean I'm telling you to eat ice cream all of the time, this is merely an example! You can even take control of this yourself and add psyllium powder when baking! Take one teaspoon of psyllium (like Metamucil or organic Psyllium powder) twice a day in water or add it to your shakes, oatmeal, or yogurt. Avoid taking psyllium or fiber before and after your resistance training as fiber slows down the absorption and insulin spike of your food which you WANT so you can supply proper nutrients as fast as possible to repair your tissue.

146) SWISS CHARD!

Swiss chard, along with spinach and beets, belong to the chenopod family which are naturally high in vitamins A, C and E, manganese and zinc. Eating Swiss chard will bring you a TON of antioxidants and anti-inflammatory benefits. It also contains magnesium and vitamin K1 which will help towards bone strength!

147) CABBAGE!

Cabbage is one of the cheapest yet most effective options when eating on a diet. The benefits that it brings to your diet are endless and there is no real excuse not to add them in. Cabbage is rich in vitamins A and C as well as many phytonutrients which can help to prevent colon, breast and prostate cancer. Cabbage also boasts a wealth of anti-inflammatory nutrients and just one serving can give you 85% of you daily vitamin K requirements! Cabbage should be eaten as CLOSE to raw as possible, over cooking or burning cabbage can remove a significant amount of nutrients and therefore benefits (the reasons why we are eating them in the first place).

Bok choy is often called 'Chinese white cabbage' and is FULL of benefits for your health. Firstly, it is rich in vitamin C and K but it also holds the highest level of vitamin A among all the cabbages. It also contains magnesium, potassium, calcium as well as others and comes with just 20 CALORIES PER CUP! Bok choy is a great option when wanting to lose weight because it fills you up due to its high fiber content!

148) COLLARD GREENS!
Collards greens are closely related to kale and as a result, offer very similar nutritional benefits. Collard greens are rich in vitamin K and help to lower 'oxidative stress' in your cells when fighting inflammation. They have also been PROVEN to prevent cancerous cells from growing and sometimes even forming in the first place.

149) BEETS!
Beets have always been popular for people on a diet because they help detoxify the body and help give you energy. This is accomplished by providing nitric oxide, opening your blood vessels, and providing more energy for your mitochondria to work efficiently both at rest and when working out. Beets are rich in vitamin C, fiber and vital minerals such as potassium and manganese. They also contain folate, the B vitamin, which helps prevent birth defects. Drinking beet juice is known to reduce blood sugar levels in just HOURS! Oh and beets are also thought to be an aphrodisiac! Just don't freak out when your excrements are RED!

150) KIMCHI!
This is a traditional dish from Korea that will help to detoxify insecticides due to lactic acid bacteria! The dish mainly uses fermented vegetables along with chili peppers, garlic and scallions. You should include a number of fermented foods in your diet so you can maximize all the different benefits that they each hold!

151) BONE BROTH!

The thought of using bones to make a healthy broth does sound strange, I will give you that, but it can be FANTASTIC for healing your gut; bone broth is known to contain both anti-inflammatory and gut-healing properties. Many allergies and problems with the immune system are caused by a 'leaky gut' and a good bone broth will help to fix this problem!

Try this recipe for Chicken Bone Broth:

Makes a nutrient-dense, mild flavored broth you can use in soups or sauces. This is a very simple recipe so you can add seasoning later on for whatever type of meal you use it for.

Chicken bones from a healthy source (1-2 carcasses leftover chicken bones)

- ✓ 2 chicken feet for extra gelatin (optional)
- ✓ 2 tablespoons Organic Apple Cider Vinegar
- ✓ 2 bay leaves (dried)
- ✓ 2 stalk of celery, 2 large carrots chopped in pieces

Optional: 1 bunch of parsley, ¾ inch-1 inch long piece of ginger, 6-8 cloves of garlic, 1 tablespoon of sea salt, 1 teaspoon of peppercorn, and additional herbs or spices to taste.

Directions: Place the bones in a large crock pot with all of the ingredients.

Pour (filtered) water over the bones and add the vinegar and bay leaves. Place in crockpot on low for 24 hours, strain and enjoy!

152) MORINGA!

Moringa is a fiber rich plant that originates from India and can be a great addition to our diet. Moringa contains isothiocyanates, and is proven to help prevent h.pylori infection, which can ultimately lead to ulcers, acid reflux and even gastric cancer. Moringa can be used the same way as spinach; you can eat it raw, cooked or steamed; benefiting from many vitamins and minerals that are in the leaves!

153) OVERNIGHT OATS FOR BREAKFAST!

This is one of my favorite hacks for a healthy breakfast, snack, or perfect pre or post workout meal. Here's how you do it:

- ✓ In a mason jar, glass container, or bowl, add a serving of quick cook oats (generally half cup dry).
- ✓ Add cinnamon for some sweetness, a serving of chia seeds, a mashed up banana, blueberries (or any other fruit), and a serving or two of your favorite protein powder.
- ✓ Add a cup of cashew milk (or any milk of your choosing) and mix ingredients so it's a little runny as the chia seeds will absorb the liquid.
- ✓ Place in the refrigerator for a couple of hours (or overnight) and enjoy this nutritious meal!
- ✓ I also like to add nuts and/or pumpkin seeds right before eating for some added crunch and nutrients.

154) ALOE VERA!

Aloe vera helps to absorb ingested nutrients and aids in strengthening your gut lining to prevent any leakages. Take the 'meat' out of the aloe and add it to juices and smoothies. You can also add it to your water (infuse flavors overnight)! It is slightly bitter so add some lemon, lime, or fruit with it, or mix the gel in salad dressings. Also, aloe releases a lot of water, has a less slimy texture, and has a milder flavor when it is cooked (steaming or poaching is best). You can also buy pure aloe gel (not the green lotion with the cartoon sun on it), but the pure (edible) aloe from a nutritional store.

155) TUMERIC TO AID JOINTS!

Turmeric, the curry spice, has actually been proven to help those with joint issues. Curcumin, which is the main ingredient in the spice, possesses anti-inflammatory and anti-arthritic properties! Turmeric is also known to fight free radicals, improve brain function, and has been shown in studies to help with depression [11]. You can add turmeric to your eggs, soups, roasted vegetables, in your morning tea, or smoothie (it's also available in capsules).

156) SPROUTS!

Sprouts are a superfood and will be a great addition to your diet! Sprouts are one of the most nutrient-dense foods that you will find, they are inexpensive and do not take much time or room to grow. They provide great support for cell regeneration, provide your body with much needed nutrients, antioxidants and minerals, and also have an 'alkalizing effect' on our bodies which can preserve muscle tissue, increase cognition, and reduce blood pressure [13]. Many tumors are acidic so sprouts can help to reduce the risk of these occurring!

157) WILD-CAUGHT SALMON!

'Wild-caught' is absolutely vital with this one! The increased amount of grain feed in a farmed environment can mean farmed raised salmon have up to 50% LESS omega-3 fats; omega-3's are the main reasons we are told to eat salmon in the first place! If you are not sure whether your salmon is wild-caught and not farmed, look for 'Alaskan salmon' or 'sockeye' as neither one of these are allowed to be farmed, ensuring you receive the full benefits from this tasty meal! Take note, since most people have caught on to the notion that 'Atlantic' means farmed raised, some establishments switched to the term 'Norwegian', which is also farmed raised!

158) CHOICE RATHER THAN CHANCE!

Our bodies are constantly working to maintain a healthy pH balance of around 7.35; where 0 is completely acidic and 14 is completely alkaline. The standard American diet contains 'foods' that are more acidic, whereas as fruits and vegetables are more alkaline. So help balance our bodies and reap the health benefits: lowered cancer risk, better digestion, better sleep, and keeping illness and infection at bay [13]!

159) SAGE FOR YOUR MEMORY!

The word sage comes from the Latin word 'salvere' which literally means 'to save'. Sage has many healing properties and was even used as an attempt to prevent the plague many years ago. Sage has also been linked with brain function and memory; the tasty herb inhibits the breakdown of acetylcholine which is a chemical messenger in the brain. Sage can therefore be a massive benefit to those who suffer from Alzheimer's in the preservation of brain function AND memory!

160) HOLY BASIL!

Holy basil is a sacred herb, originally from India that is different to regular basil. Holy basil can prevent the growth of bacteria and provide a significant boost to the immune system. Holy basil is also being studied further for its blood pressure and anxiety reduction.

161) FENUGREEK!

The first question I am sure that you have is 'What the HECK is that?' as it is a lesser known herb. Fenugreek was originally used in Ayurveda medicine as it was known for enhancing libido and masculinity. Despite research, those findings have been inconclusive. However, Fenugreek does have a big impact on blood sugar levels as it contains 4-hydroxyisoleucine; which improves the function of the hormone insulin leading to a lower body fat and reduced blood sugar levels. Add it to soups, salads, or even in your tea (it's great for digestion as well).

162) ROSEMARY IS HEALTHY!

The main ingredient in rosemary is called rosmarinic acid which suppresses allergy responses as well as nasal congestion. Even as little as 50mg is thought to suppress allergy symptoms! Sprinkle rosemary in soups, salads, or even on toasted whole grain bread.

163) GARLIC TO STAY WELL!

Garlic's distinct smell is caused by a compound called allicin which can actually offer us some handy health benefits. If you suffer from regular colds, adding more garlic to your diet should do the trick! It is also thought to lead to better heart health, lower cholesterol and blood pressure! Wow that clove of garlic really packs a punch and of course, keeps vampires away!

164) SQUASH SKIN DAMAGE!

Butternut squash is a GREAT addition to your diet because it contains carotenoids; which are powerful antioxidants that work hard at reducing skin cell damage!

165) SUPER GREENS TO THE RESCUE!

As stated several times most of us do not get the recommended amount of vegetables in our daily diet, but SUPER GREENS can truly be your HERO! Many foods provide a complex range of nutrients, and super greens are considered one of the best sources of nutrition available! The grocery store is full of greens like spinach, lettuce, chard, and kale, but look for the word *super green! It* refers to a small group of greens from the algae and cereal grass families including: spirulina, chlorella, wheatgrass, and barley grass [14]. So don't worry; you don't have to be a hippy to reap the benefits of super greens!

- ✓ **SPIRULINA** – Spirulina is a form of blue algae that forms from warm fresh water bodies. Spirulina boasts 4g of protein per tablespoon and is extremely high in percentage of complete protein (65-71% complete protein compared to beef, which is only 22%, and lentils which has 26%). In addition to the protein benefits, spirulina has been shown to boost the immune system, improve digestion, reduce fatigue, build endurance, cleanse the body, boost energy levels, control appetite, maintain healthy cardiovascular function, support the liver and kidneys, reduce inflammation, and lessen symptoms of allergies. There are many types of spirulina available so it is important to do your homework before making a purchase. Choose an organic spirulina from a reputable source. Spirulina comes in capsules, tablets, powders and flakes. The recommended daily dose is typically between three to five grams. Make sure to increase your intake of spring or filtered water when taking spirulina to help it absorb into your system. Fun fact: NASA conducted studies on Spirulina as a potential food for space travel. The goal of space travel is to provide the astronauts with foods that are in rich in nutrients but don't take up much space. **NASA found that 1 kg of Spirulina had the same nutrients found in about 1,000 kg of assorted vegetables!**

- ✓ **CHLORELLA** – Chlorella is blue green algae similar to Spirulina but closer to a plant than an algae. Chlorella contains chlorophyll, attributing to its green color, but it also provides many health benefits. Chlorophyll can improve immunity, alkalinity, and inflammation; it can even fight bad breath, excellent! Chlorella also helps with detoxification, digestion, energy, and provides important vitamins, minerals and amino acids.

✓ **WHEATGRASS** – Wheatgrass is among the youngest of all cereal grass. Wheatgrass is high in chlorophyll, protein and concentrated nutrients such as Vitamins A, C, E, Iron, Calcium, magnesium, and amino acids. Wheatgrass is GLUTEN FREE because it is cut and used before the grain actually forms. Wheat grass has been shown to renew tissue, purify the liver, and contains 70% chlorophyll which is an important blood builder and has even been shown to help slow down the aging process. You can grow wheatgrass in your home, take a wheatgrass shot (the drinkable kind), or buy powdered wheatgrass and add it to your water, fresh juices, or smoothies.

✓ **BARLEY GRASS** – Barley grass refers to the young soft green shoots which crop up on the Barley plant. Barley is a nutrient rich super food loaded with vitamins like A, B1(thiamine), B2 (riboflavin), B3 (niacin), B6, folate, C (ascorbic acid), E (alpha- tocopherol) and vitamin K (phylloquinone), electrolytes, and other essential minerals. Barley grass also detoxifies the body by getting rid of harmful heavy metals such as zinc, copper, and selenium, which can lead to behavior problems in kids. Barley is also known to increase your immune system and is known to regenerate cells. Another amazing benefit of barley is that it can help fight addiction with the presence of glutamic acid; which inhibits the craving for harmful materials such as alcohol, coffee, nicotine, drugs and even sugary sweets. Barley grass can be consumed as a juice extracted from the cereal grass sprouts or in the form of green powder.*If you are sensitive to gluten stay away from Barley products as they may contain gluten.

✓ **POWDER UP!** – Now that you know the power of supergreens why not get them all in one bang for your buck?! There are a number of super greens powders that provide all of your essential vitamins, minerals, nutrients, and electrolytes in one serving. If you want a little extra sweetness you can even find them in a variety of flavors including dark chocolate which goes great with your protein shakes or greens smoothies! Some powders even add a full complement of your fruits and veggies.

166) DRINK YOUR VITAMINS!

Most of us lack color in our diets and with a lack of color often indicates a lack of vitamins. If the thought of taking a green powder has you feeling, well, green, then opt for a liquid multivitamin. Look for a brand that doesn't add any sugar; add it to your water, smoothie, protein shake, or simply take a shot of it every day!

167) PROTEIN WITH EVERY MEAL!

Protein should be ingested with each meal if possible. Some concerns have arisen about elevated protein consumption placing stress on the kidneys. However, if you are adequately hydrated and are consuming ample quantities of fiber through moderate to high consumption of unrefined carbohydrate foods, you should not place excessive strain on the kidneys at all [33]. As mentioned, I would prefer you to get your protein through clean sources if possible. Organic foods are usually more expensive, but if you are able to afford it the extra expense is worthwhile.

168) MAKE YOUR OWN PROTEIN ICE CREAM!

Oh, there is nothing better than treating yourself to some delicious ice cream! Maybe you do 'deserve' a treat, but if you make a habit of it, it's likely to go straight to your love handles! Try my Protein Ice Cream recipe that I absolutely LOVE! Here's what you do: in a blender, or NutriBullet (seriously, these things are amazing and I'm not even being paid to say that!), add a cup of ice and your favorite milk or milk substitute (like coconut milk, almond milk, or my favorite cashew milk). Add a serving of your favorite low sugar protein powder and some fruit like berries or a banana. Place a tablespoon or two of any organic unsweetened nut butter and cinnamon to taste. Blend until creamy and add some crunch with mixed nuts, pumpkin seeds, sunflower seeds, or unsweetened shredded coconut. If you want a thicker consistency place in the freezer for 10-15 minutes and enjoy! This will save you all of the guilt, several hundred calories, spare your waistline, and satisfy your sweet tooth all while enjoying a delicious snack that's good for you! This entire treat is around 300 calories (depends on your protein powder), packs 25-50 grams of protein, and is very low in sugar! Enjoy!

169) BUCKWHEAT BEFORE WORKOUT!

Buckwheat is a fruit seed that digests slowly and helps fat-burning as well as increasing endurance!

170) PEPPERMINT IS A BRAIN FOOD!

The next time you are struggling to concentrate, have some peppermint! Peppermint is proven to increase the amount of oxygen in your blood, which means more oxygen is going to your brain, allowing you to focus!

171) 'ENGINEER' QUICK PROTEIN ABSORPTION!

For most meals, I suggest you consume whole foods as opposed to engineered proteins; however the pre and post workout meals are an exception. If you are time restricted, engineered protein foods such as shakes may be a good substitute for regular foods. The reason I love engineered proteins such as those found in shakes for the pre and post workout meals is that they are rapidly absorbed in the bloodstream, available for almost immediate use by the body. They are digested far more quickly than whole foods and are useful before a high intensity workout, and after the crushing effect of an intense workout on the body.

Alcohol Hacks

172) Skip the BOOZE AND LOSE!

Liquid courage, Uncle Jack, party in a bottle. These are all names commonly used when it comes to describing our national pastime…drinking. Alcohol is the main attraction at most sporting events, parties, and gatherings, but are we aware of how the first sip of alcohol affects your bodies internally…and eventually your waistline? We all have seen the commercials touting low calorie, low carb, no guilt alcoholic beverages – the ones we can drink while keeping our ripped abs intact. What these commercials don't tell you is the sneaky tricks happening inside that will immediately halt the hard work and reverse progress made in your health journey. Several aspects about alcohol are becoming more prevalent among the masses. Alcohol is full of "empty" calories. Stay away from mixers with loads of sweeteners. Be sure to eat something before you drink. And while these are all somewhat true, they barely scratch the surface.

Below are the *not so ordinary* ways alcohol will wreak havoc on your waistline and your health:

✓ **Alcohol & Blood Sugar.** Contrary to what we'd like to believe, alcohol is poisonous to the body. Once consumed, the body makes every effort to rid itself of the poison. What's more, alcohol directly affects your bodies' ability to maintain healthy blood sugar levels by inhibiting the secretion of insulin. The insulin hormone is secreted whenever the body is introduced to a component that's processed as a sugar (think carbohydrates, desserts, fruit, etc). If your body is unable to stabilize blood sugar levels because of alcohol's effect on insulin, it will store those extra sugars in your body in the form of body fat! Aside from decreasing insulin sensitivity, alcohol can also lower the body's blood sugar when consumed on an empty stomach, leading to hypoglycemia (low blood sugar levels). Working out naturally lowers blood sugar, so if you have as few as two drinks in a day and then engage in physical activity, energy levels will plummet. This lack of energy will be a detriment to your fitness goals and possibly cause even more life threatening health problems…aside from the possibility of passing out on the treadmill.

✓ **Alcohol & Caloric Intake.** The body requires a certain amount of calories to maintain a certain weight, and that's based on height, weight, and gender (called your basal metabolic rate, BMR (refer to hack#36)). A surplus of calories will increase your weight because your body can't utilize those calories as energy, but rather stores them as fat. In addition to the extra calories and sugar introduced to the body through alcohol, drinking during a meal has been shown to increase the amount of calories you consume by 20 percent. All told, the calories from the alcohol combined with the food calories in a typical meal, the average individual will consume 33 percent more calories in a meal with alcohol than without. The "beer belly" is very real. In fact, a study of more than 3,000 men who drank on a regular basis had excess amounts of belly fat leading to an increased risk of Type 2 diabetes. When we drink, our hunger increases and with a lowered inhibition we are more likely to crave bad foods late at night and make bad food choices… a cocktail recipe for disaster!

✓ **Alcohol & Testosterone.** Another risk of alcohol consumption is a decreased level of testosterone. Testosterone is responsible for muscle growth, energy, sex drive, and helps increase metabolism. When consumed, alcohol disrupts the release of free testosterone. Think of free testosterone as the fuel in your gas tank – it should be available for immediate use to the body, which isn't the case when alcohol is involved. Further, the hops in beer are known to be extremely estrogenic. An elevated level of estrogen in a man will decrease overall testosterone; hops are even being studied to lower the symptoms of hot flashes in post-menopausal women.

✓ **Alcohol & Circadian Rhythm.** Alcohol affects the body's natural circadian rhythm. When a person doesn't get a good night's sleep, it can't produce the growth hormone responsible for bone and muscle growth. The result can be inflammation, slowed muscle repair, and increased hunger the next day. Then, you guessed it, you're more apt to eat too many calories and derail your weight loss progress.

✓ **Alcohol & Metabolism.** Alcohol and the body's metabolic function don't mix. Too often, the focus is on the calories, carbs, and sugars in alcohol while overlooking how the alcohol is broken down. Once alcohol is consumed, the body makes it a priority to get it out, which might seem like a good thing. But it's not. Since the body can't metabolize alcohol, it will put the brakes on metabolizing other nutrients, protein, carbohydrates, and fat. The body simply registers the foreign substance in your body and won't break down any calories, making you more likely to store fat. Once you stop drinking, alcohol leaves the body at about .01% per hour, so if your blood alcohol content (BAC) is .08 (legal limit) it will take you eight hours to get all of the alcohol out of your system. Only then can your body begin metabolizing fat. Don't think that coffee, a cold shower, or greasy food will help you get rid of the toxins in your body. Time is the ONLY thing that will help.

173) ALCOHOL DAMAGE CONTROL!

Now that the risks of alcohol consumption have been identified, you probably won't ever drink again, right? Wrong. As a realist, it's important to identify how to responsibly consume alcohol while minimizing damage to your waistline here's how:

✓ Never drink on an empty stomach.

✓ Don't drink before a meal; you're more likely to consume added calories.

✓ Drink one glass of water for every alcoholic beverage.

✓ Limit the amount of alcohol consumed in the evening, when it's harder for your body to break it down.

✓ Don't drink sugary mixers. Instead, stick with water, soda water, or fresh juice.

✓ Stick to a glass or two of wine. Just because it has beneficial properties doesn't mean you can drink the whole bottle.

✓ Don't. Do. Shots. It's harder to monitor your alcohol intake. (If you can somehow manage to just do shots, avoid the mixers, and limit yourself, then go ahead, but don't say I didn't warn you!)

✓ Set a limit, and stick to it. You'll feel better the next morning.

✓ Drink slower. Enjoy it more and, hopefully, drink less.

✓ Talk to yourself! Ask yourself if a third drink is worth undoing the hard work you've been putting into to achieving your fitness and nutrition goals. Odds are, it's not.

174) BE CHOOSY WHEN CONSUMING ALCOHOL!

Know what the best and worst options are:

✓ **Best:** White or Red Wine. Red or white wine contains roughly 100 to 120 calories per glass (assuming that's a standard 5oz glass, research from Cornell says people over pour by about 12 %!) White wine typically contains fewer carbs than red, which makes a small difference in terms of calories, but red wine is richer in antioxidants. In fact a 2014 study in *The Journal of Nutritional Biochemistry* stated that red wine's Ellagic acids delay the growth of fat cells while slowing the development of new ones (don't use this as an excuse to down the entire bottle) [25].

✓ **Best:** Liquor is quicker, ha! When you need to watch your calories straight liquor is one of your best options you have. There isn't a huge difference between proof of hard liquors. They all have around the same amount of calories and carbohydrates. For example, a shot of 86-proof whiskey contains 105 calories and a shot of 80-proof vodka contains 97. What you do need to consider is that the sweeter the liquor the higher the sugar content (and the higher the calories and carbs). Avoid flavored vodkas, spiced rums, and anything else that tastes sweet, if it tastes sweet odds are there is extra sugar in it! Go for the plain version of your favorite liquor and have it on the rocks, neat, with water, soda water, or fresh squeezed lemon or lime. These improve the taste without the calories!

✓ **Best:** Vermouth. Vermouth is a fortified wine generally served in Europe with a higher alcohol content and infused with spices and herbs. A 1.5-ounce serving contains a minimal 64 calories with about 15 to 18 percent alcohol. Research has shown that it's packed with polyphenol compounds which may promote healthy weight loss, in moderation [26]! Vermouth is commonly used in a Martini as well as a Manhattan. Don't use the polyphenol excuse with these two mixed drinks as you will add a lot more calories and sugar to your "healthy" vermouth.

✓ **Best:** With fewer calories and carbs many light beers contain 90 to 100 calories per 12 ounces, while extra-light beers pack about 55 to 65. Now I know what you are thinking, "I can drink more beers now!" Don't use that as an excuse to have more beers than you typically would, or could undo all of your hard work! Be careful with light brews because they tend to have a higher percentage of their calories coming from alcohol compared to standard brews. Budweiser Select 55 has 88.2 percent of its calories from alcohol, compared to Bud Light at 74.1 percent, and regular Budweiser at 66.9 percent calories, take it slow or your belly will show!

✓ **Worst:** Cocktails with tons of Sugar! Margaritas, Long Island Iced Teas, and the myriad of drinks served with an umbrella have more calories than a large order of French Fries! One of the worst parts of these drinks is they are so loaded with sugar, it overwhelms your body so all its left to do is store the sugar in your drink as fat! Stay away from the sweet cocktails if you want a sweet figure.

✓ **Worst:** Craft Beers. The past several years have been booming with new craft beers to suck down in your local pub but they may do more harm than good! The high alcohol content in much of these craft beers also creates a high calorie and carb content. The more alcohol in a beer means more calories;

as 1 gram of alcohol (within the beverage) equals 7 calories. Some of the beers can contain as much as 450 plus calories in an 18% alcohol bottle, wow, might as well have a juicy burger!

I'm not telling you not to drink; I simply want you to know what is going into your body, and more importantly, what is going on inside your body once you chug that beer.

Fat Burning Hacks

Don't spend hundreds on pre-packaged fat burning products, especially since some supplement companies include a "proprietary blend" in their ingredients which can be anything they want to add, yikes! Listed below are some supplements that can help give you a fat burning boost. Be sure to only choose one supplement combo at a time. Overdoing supplements, especially those meant to increase your metabolism, may leave you feeling ill (some can experience rapid heart rate, anxiety, and trouble sleeping from too many stimulants). Before taking any of the following supplements consult with your health care provider.

175) GREEN TEA EXTRACT AND CAFFEINE!
Both of these ingredients can often be found in costly fat-burner supplements. As the price of these can cost more than food for a week; and yes, you need to EAT to lose weight, don't get any funny ideas! Buying these ingredients separately will be a fraction of the cost! Caffeine works to increase fat-burning during both rest and exercise; caffeine is great at binding to fat cells and increasing the removal of fat while preventing more fat from being stored. Green tea also contains catechins, which are compounds that increase the amount of fat that can be burned. Try between 100-300mg in pill form of caffeine, or a cup of coffee (half this amount if you aren't used to caffeine), mixed in with around 600-800mg of green tea extract in the morning and then again an hour before your workout. If it is your rest day, you can still have a second dose in the afternoon, just make sure it's not close to bed time as you will have problems sleeping!

176) MAKE YOUR OWN FAT BURNING DRINK!

Try my Renovation Tea. Renovation tea can help a sluggish metabolism which is often caused by inflammation. Many of the ingredients in this tea help to not only reduce inflammation, they increase blood flow and regulate blood sugar. This recipe uses a few simple ingredients and can easily be made at home. Directions: bring a gallon of water to a boil; add about 15-20 bags of Matcha Green Tea as it has been shown to aid in cancer prevention, has anti-aging properties and contributes to weight loss. Add three lemons (sliced) and three limes (sliced). Lemons and limes have vitamin C and their potassium and citric acid offer numerous benefits from flushing out toxins to aiding in digestion. Once the sliced citrus has been added place a few slices of fresh ginger root (ginger aids in digestion, reduces inflammation, and increases the metabolism). Depending on your preference of sizzle and spice, add one to four dried red hot chili peppers to further increase your metabolic rate due to the capsaicin. A few cinnamon sticks or a tablespoon of powdered cinnamon are added to the mixture for an antioxidant boost and anti-inflammatory benefits. Also add a slice of turmeric (curcumin is the primary pharmacological agent in the spice) or some turmeric tea bags as it aids in reducing inflammation, it's an excellent source of phytonutrients, helps digest fats, reduces gas and bloating (bonus), decreases congestion, relieves joint pain, reduces joint swelling, and helps range of motion. After the concoction has had a chance to stand for one to two hours, it is time to strain into a refrigerator safe container. Take a glass of Renovation Tea every morning, before a workout, or anytime you need a pick me up! Be careful before bedtime though as there is some caffeine from the green tea (you may also use caffeine free green tea bags).

177) GINGER AND RED PEPPER!

Make it easier on yourself and eat these foods to increase your metabolism. The red pepper aids fat-burning by using a double pronged attack; it significantly reduces your hunger so you will see your calorie intake reduce nicely but it also contains a chemical, capsaicin, which increases your metabolic rate and fat-burning as it raises your levels of norepinephrine (increases energy output by your body). Ginger can increase your lactic acid production in your muscles which will stimulate growth hormone release and lipolysis (breakdown of fats) thus leading to fat-loss.

178) SESAMIN AND TTA!

Sesamin is a strong antioxidant and a fantastic fat-burner! It is found in foods like flaxseed, wheat bran, pumpkin seeds, and sesame seeds of course! Sesamin works by activating a specific muscle receptor, PPAR alpha, found in the heart, muscles and liver cells. PPAR alpha turns on genes that decrease fat storage and increase fat-burning! Tetradecylthioacetic acid (TTA) is a fatty acid that contains sulphur which means that it cannot be burned for fuel; instead it regulates the burning and storage of dietary fats! Try combining 250-1000mg of Sesamin and 250-1000mg of TTA with breakfast, lunch AND dinner!

179) SELENIUM, ZINC AND CALCIUM!

These three minerals will not only help to keep you healthy on the inside, they will also help you STAY lean! Selenium is vital for the production of thyroid hormones, without which our metabolism would suffer! Zinc is also important as being low in this mineral can severely impact our thyroid hormone production which makes it harder to lose body fat. Finally, calcium helps to regulate and suppress the hormone calcitriol, which causes the body to produce fat AND prevents fat breakdown. Calcium also reduces the amount of fat that is absorbed by your intestines! You should take 200-400mcg of selenium with 1000mg of calcium DAILY with your food. Zinc is slightly harder to consume so the most effective way is to take a ZMA supplement on an empty stomach before bed. This will provide you with around 30mg of zinc.

180) CARNITINE AND FORSKOLIN!

This combination allows fat to be accessed and then be burned for energy while you exercise, maximizing your fat-burning! Forskolin works by activating an enzyme whose main job is to create another enzyme that increases the ability of stored fat to be released into the bloodstream. Carnitine then helps that same fat to be used for fuel and energy. Try 300-500mg of Forskolin and 2-3 grams of Carnitine with breakfast, pre-workout meals AND post-workout meals.

181) ARGININE AND GLUTAMINE!

Both of these are amino acids with outstanding fat-burning qualities that are exemplified when combined together! Arginine is well known for boosting nitric oxide levels which, amongst other things, makes it an extremely helpful fat-burner as it enhances lipolysis (breakdown of fat). With the increased metabolic burn (achieved from the glutamine), the 'freed' fat is more likely to be burned for fuel! You can take 2-3 grams of arginine and 1-2 grams of glutamine up to 3 times a day (or the recommended dosage on the bottle); preferably 30-60 minutes before breakfast, before and after working out, and before bed. Foods that contain arginine include: nuts, legumes, sunflower seeds, and dairy products. Natural sources of glutamine are: meat, poultry, seafood, dairy products, lentils, peas, beans, and cabbage.

182) YES WHEY!

Now of course protein powders have been used for years when attempting to stimulate muscle growth but not many people know that they can also encourage weight loss! Whey powder SIGNIFICANTLY increases the production of 'hunger-blunting' hormones which means that you will feel fuller longer. For example, if you were to have a whey protein shake before a buffet, it is highly likely that you would eat less than you would have done without the whey protein. As a result, you consume fewer calories each day and shed the pounds. Try consuming a shake containing 20 grams of whey IMMEDIATELY before a workout. After a workout, take a shake that contains 20-30g.

183) FISH OIL AND CLA!

Last, but by no means least, is the great combination of fish oil and conjugated linoleic acid (CLA)! A long time ago, everyone thought that foods containing fat were bad for us and so we were advised to stay away from healthy foods like almonds, salmon, olive oil, etc. However, we now know that the right fats actually benefit our bodies, especially omega-3s, found in fish oil. Omega-3 fatty acids are now known to be an important component to burning fat as it helps to prevent dietary fats from becoming stored body fats! Couple this with CLA (naturally found in meat and dairy) and you have a great combination as CLA will inhibit lipoprotein lipase; which is an enzyme that picks up fat from circulation and helps to store it as body fat (we don't want that)! Try to take around 2 grams of each at breakfast, lunch and dinner!

Nutrition Plan: 10-Day Remodel Detox

184) 10 DAY REMODEL DETOX!

Liquid detoxes, cleanses, and strange magic potions. There are all sorts of fad diets available to us nowadays, so we never know what foods are actually best for OUR bodies. We hear that gluten is bad; along with soy, dairy, tofu, fat, sugar, the list goes on and on; but the truth is everyone is different and until you know what affects you, you will never truly know what foods aren't good for you personally. We have one body in this life and ONE chance to live a healthy energetic life. Why do we still feel so inspired to ruin it and not look after it? With my 10-Day Remodel Detox, we will be slowly removing foods that are known to be harmful to our bodies until they are eventually out of our diet! Most detoxes and diets tend to suggest removal straight away and you are left feeling so hungry; you eat less, consume fewer calories and therefore have no energy. This WILL NOT happen if you follow the 10-Day Remodel Detox. It is vital that we carry on consuming enough calories to get by; we will just be changing how we get those calories!

The main idea of this 'remodel' is to get our bodies back to basics. We throw so many unhealthy foods into our system that we no longer know how our body responds to each food, let alone what they are supposed to do within our bodies! During this remodel, you will allow yourself the chance to figure out what is bothering you by taking these foods out one by one and then slowly reintroducing them back into your diet to truly be in tune with yourself. This remodel will help to set your body back to homeostasis (equilibrium) so that we can begin to feel the full effects of our nutrition.

FOODS THAT WILL BE REMOVED DURING THE REMODEL:

Gluten – A little known fact about gluten, is that it is derived from the Latin word 'glue'; yes, GLUE! It is a protein found in grains like wheat, barley, and rye that provide elasticity, shape, and chewy texture to our foods. Removing gluten from your diet can benefit your body greatly. You are actually less likely to get cravings for sugary foods because most foods that contain gluten are generally loaded with refined carbohydrates and will be processed by your body as sugar to store as fat.

Dairy Products – Many studies and tests have been run with people dropping dairy from their diet and it is becoming more and more popular because of how good they felt once they made the change. Dairy products are known for causing inflammation and constipation; surely it is worth it to reduce the likelihood of those two occurring!

Caffeinated Drinks – Everybody drinks caffeine, right? But as I said before, the idea of this remodel is to return our bodies to equilibrium and to start to feel the effects of what we consume as we reintroduce them back into our diets. Caffeine can have a hugely negative impact on our insulin resistance, our sleep, our blood pressure and more!

Red Meats – As well as damaging your cells, red meats are also infamous for their high cholesterol levels and insulin resistance as they are filled with hormones and antibiotics!

Finally…Refined Sugars – 'but they taste so good!' There is a reason for this…they are terrible for our health! Our taste buds have been changed and ruined by refined sugars! We used to be happy with fruit; they used to fulfill our sweet tooth, but this is no longer the case due to the rise of refined sugars. Artificial sweeteners and excess sugar can cause diabetes, weight problems, inflammation, blood pressure problems AND MORE! Let's go back to basics and remove them from our diet!

The 10 Day Remodel Detox Plan isn't your average "detox" where you starve yourself for days and drink beverages that make your stomach churn. This is a program to get you on the right track to health while actually EATING FOOD!

Days 1 - 7 reflect an elimination plan that builds on recommendations from the days prior. Once a food category has been eliminated, do NOT add it back until advised. Your healthcare provider may make additional dietary suggestions or limitations. Always use organic foods when possible. You will be eating or having a shake every 2-3 hours.

SIMPLE EXERCISE - Strenuous or prolonged exercise should be reduced during the program to allow your body to cleanse and rejuvenate more effectively. You can gain benefit from walking 30 minutes 3 times a week, (if you are a seasoned fitness enthusiast light weight training/cardio 3 times per week). You should follow the advice of your healthcare provider.

STRESS MANAGEMENT - Adequate stress reduction and sleep are important to the success of the program. Your body is recharging and regenerating - help it by getting adequate rest!

EATING PLAN - A modified elimination diet rich in vitamins, minerals, and phyto-nutrients reduces the allergen and toxin load, helping the body to detoxify efficiently. For best results, carefully adhere to the Dietary Guidelines. Foods that are not found under Food Choices should NOT be eaten, unless discussed with your healthcare provider. Most detoxes are extremely low in protein, I recommend you get a vegan protein powder to add to your recommended nightly shakes. You can find a good list of vegan protein powder on Amazon: For vegan protein powders I'm partial to the Vega or Orgain brand; any will do as long as there isn't any added sugar or preservatives. In general, most vegan protein powders are good (they can also be found at your local health food store, GNC, Vitamin World, etc.). According to the Institute of Health, men need about 56 grams of protein per day and women need 46 grams per day. Try to at least get the minimum amount required in a day on the remodel. Most Vegan protein powders have about 25 grams per serving.

If you can't get a vegan protein you may add a serving of cold water fish (such as mackerel, haddock, tuna, cod, salmon and trout), or organic skinless chicken/turkey breast to your meal to keep the protein content up. Having 2 fist size servings of protein will meet your minimum requirement for each day.

PREPARATION PRIOR TO STARTING 10 DAY REMODEL DETOX

To be successful on your program, you need to be prepared. Take time to learn what foods you will need for your program. You are more likely to stay on course if you make a shopping list and plan your meals for the week ahead and get rid of the foods that you have in the house that are not allowed on the plan and may tempt you. To save time you can make several servings at the same time for future meals. To save money, look for sales at Whole Foods, Green Wise, Mariano's, Trader Joe's or Costco stores on organic foods and stock up and freeze what you can't use immediately. Even "ordinary" grocery stores now carry organic foods. Purchase all organic/all natural products if possible; especially produce and meat/poultry/fish. Remember to wash all of your fruits and vegetables properly.

Shopping List- You may have lots of these ingredients, or you may not have any, not to worry, prepare for your success! This is NOT an exhaustive list of ingredients and you may end up having to pick up some more ingredients as the plan goes on and change the recommended meals for some of the days. Depending on the meals you choose you may need more or less of these ingredients. Go through each day to see what meals you will be likely to eat and then cross check this general shopping list.

✓ Almond Butter
✓ Apples
✓ Apple Cider Vinegar
✓ Avocado
✓ Baby Peas
✓ Bananas (4-5)
✓ Bell Pepper
✓ Berries (fresh or frozen blueberries, raspberries, strawberries, etc.)
✓ Broccoli
✓ Brown Rice
✓ Butternut Squash
✓ Carrots
✓ Celery
✓ Chicken/turkey breast
✓ Cucumber
✓ Garbanzo Beans (Chickpeas) – can substitute plain hummus
✓ Gluten Free Oatmeal
✓ Green leafy vegetables (kale. Spinach, Swiss chard, etc.)
✓ Hemp Seeds (optional)

✓ Herbs- Parsley, Dill, Cilantro, Basil or may substitute any herb of your choice
✓ Hummus
✓ Kidney/Red beans
✓ Lemons (several)
✓ Nondairy milk (Unsweetened coconut, rice, or hemp milk)
✓ Olive Oil
✓ Onions
✓ Pears
✓ Pineapple (fresh or frozen)
✓ Raw mixed nuts (no peanuts)
✓ Raw sunflower and pumpkin seeds
✓ Spices-Cinnamon, Cayenne, Cumin, Chili powder, Salt, Pepper
✓ Quinoa
✓ Scallions
✓ Sweet potatoes
✓ Vegan Protein Powder

DAY 1

Today you are ELIMINATING:

- ✓ Refined sugars - anything with added sucrose, high fructose corn syrup, or alcohol (cakes, cookies, candies, pastries, beer, wine, liquor). - This category will be tough for most to eliminate, but remember to stay the course one day and one meal at a time!

- ✓ Caffeinated drinks (soda, coffee, tea). - You may have Green Tea (don't overdo it) or herbal caffeine free teas.

- ✓ Artificial coloring, flavorings, and sweeteners (packaged & processed foods)

- ✓ Beef, lamb, pork, poultry, non-cold water fish, wild game (no red meat)

The easiest route may be simply choosing from the recipe suggestions. If you wish to develop your own recipes, keep the Dietary Guidelines in mind.

BREAKFAST	Metabolism Boosting Green Shake **AND** Gluten free Oatmeal or Cooked Quinoa Flakes **OR** Scrambled Eggs w/Veggies (see recipe below)
SNACK	Raw Veggie sticks with hummus and/or Vegan Protein in water
LUNCH	Quinoa Salad topped with Avocado Slices **OR** Mixed greens salad w/chicken breast, veggies, and walnuts (see recipe below)
SNACK	Handful of raw mixed nuts (no peanuts), Metabolism Boosting Green shake, **OR** apple with almond or cashew butter
DINNER	Berry and Coconut Smoothie (see recipe below)

RECIPES:

Metabolism Boosting Green Shake

This nutrient rich green shake will decrease inflammation and speed up your metabolism with a dash of cayenne pepper. *Directions:* Add ½ cup of fresh or frozen pineapple, 1 cup of spinach, ¼ teaspoon cayenne (less or more as you choose, be careful it's spicy!), 1 full peeled small lemon, 1 cup of cucumber with peel, and 1-2 cups of water as necessary. Blend until smooth (may add ice).

Gluten Free Oatmeal with Banana

½ -1 cup of Gluten Free Oatmeal or cooked quinoa flakes topped with ½ - 1cup of UNSWEETENED almond, coconut, hemp, or rice milk. Heat in a saucepan or microwave until desired consistency. Add sliced banana or raisins and sprinkle with cinnamon. May add berries, chia seeds, flax seeds, or mixed nuts (no peanuts) for added flavor.

Calories: 355, Carbs: 67g, Protein:9g, Fat: 6g, Fiber: 9g

Basic Salad Dressing

This recipe makes 2-3 servings. Increase recipe for multiple servings. Keep a jar in the refrigerator at work and one at home for convenience.

- ✓ ¼ cup flax seed oil (or 2 Tbsp. flax seed and 2 Tbsp. olive oil)
- ✓ 1-2 Tbsp. vinegar (apple cider, tarragon, rice, red wine, balsamic, Ume plum)
- ✓ ½ - 1 Tbsp. water
- ✓ 1 tsp Dijon-type mustard (optional), whisked in to liquid for easy mixing
- ✓ Whole or minced garlic, oregano, basil or other herbs of choice.

Mix well in a shaker jar and store any leftovers in your refrigerator

Quinoa Salad

This recipe serves 2. You may adjust as needed and/or add any leftover veggie for variety.

- ✓ ¾ cup quinoa, rinsed well
- ✓ 1 ½ cups vegetable broth or water
- ✓ 1 red bell diced pepper
- ✓ 1 cup frozen baby peas
- ✓ thawed 1/4 cup diced red onion
- ✓ 3 scallions, thinly sliced or 1 chopped shallot
- ✓ ¼ cup fresh dill, chopped
- ✓ ¼ cup parsley, chopped
- ✓ Sliced avocado (1 small)

Directions: Add quinoa to broth or water in a medium sauce pan, stir and bring to a boil. Reduce to simmer; then cover and cook 15 minutes without stirring or until liquid is absorbed. Remove ingredients from saucepan and place in a bowl. Cool slightly and toss with 1/2 cup Basic salad dressing and remaining ingredients. Adjust seasoning to taste.

May add chicken, turkey or fish. Portion size: Men 6-8oz,Women 4-6 oz. (palm size portion)

Calories per Serving: 370, Carbs: 66g Protein: 18g, Fat: 4g Fiber: 10g (w/o chicken)

Berry and Coconut Smoothie

This tasty dairy free smoothie is great for post workout, a snack, and at night to keep you full until bedtime. UNSWEETENED Coconut milk or almond milk (if you are eliminating nuts do NOT use almond milk) can be used to add healthy fat and little sugar.

- ✓ 10-12 frozen strawberries.
- ✓ 8 ounces coconut milk.
- ✓ 1 tsp almond butter.

Directions: Use frozen strawberries, blueberries, or raspberries to keep from diluting the smoothie mix (if you are eliminating nuts take out the almond butter). Blend all the ingredients in the blender until smooth.

*Add a serving or two of a Vegan protein powder if desired (about 25-30 grams of protein)

You may add sunflower or pumpkin seeds before or after for some crunch.

Calories w/o protein powder: 131g, Carbs: 13g, Protein: 3g, Fat: 8g, Fiber: 4g *Note the calorie content may vary depending on protein powder.*

DAY 2

In addition to eliminating foods listed for Day 1

ELIMINATE ALL: Dairy products and eggs

PRE-BREAKFAST	Elixir Shot (see recipe below)
BREAKFAST	Metabolism Boosting Green Shake **AND** Gluten free Oatmeal **OR** Cooked Quinoa Flakes w/ Berries (see Day 1)
SNACK	Detox Green Smoothie
LUNCH	Minestrone Soup **OR** Fruit salad w/ cinnamon (see recipe below)
SNACK	Detox Green Smoothie

DINNER	Berry Coconut Smoothie

RECIPES:

Elixir Shot

No, this isn't a shot of booze! I'm talking about my Elixir Shot! Fermented foods offer amazing digestive/immune support and the best thing is they are CHEAP, bonus! Mix lemon juice from 1 full lemon, 2 tablespoon of Apple Cider Vinegar (ACV), ½ teaspoon cinnamon, a little water if it's too bitter for you and you prefer to dilute it. Add a dash of cayenne for an added kick (optional). ACV will improve the digestion of all of the amazing superfoods you will be eating throughout your detox. The ideal amount of ACV is 2 tbsps, but play around with the mixture to see what's best for you.

*Ok, I didn't think this sounded too great when I first started doing it but I promise you it will help with your detoxification process. This Morning Elixir can be taken before any meal, not just the morning. To really give your metabolism a boost you may add a tablespoon of cinnamon and a few sprinkles of cayenne. The cinnamon will help with blood sugar regulation and inflammation and the cayenne will boost your metabolism and give you energy for the day. Be careful it's spicy!

Detox Green Smoothie

- ✓ 1 cup Kale or collard greens, firmly packed (stems removed & chopped)
- ✓ 1/2 cup loosely packed parsley leaves
- ✓ 1/2 medium apple, cored & coarsely chopped
- ✓ 1/2 medium pear, cored & coarsely chopped 3/4 cup ice (optional)
- ✓ 1 1/2 cups water

Combine all ingredients in a blender and blend until smooth. If too thick, add more water.

Calories: 142 Carbs: 35g Protein: 4g Fat: 1g Fiber: 7g

Minestrone Soup (serves 2)

You may adjust the ingredients to accommodate your desired portions.

- ✓ ½ Tbsp. olive oil
- ✓ ½ medium to large onion, chopped
- ✓ 1 ½ carrots, sliced or diced
- ✓ 1 stalks celery, diced
- ✓ 1 garlic cloves, minced
- ✓ 3 cups vegetable stock (low sodium)
- ✓ ½ bay leaf
- ✓ 1/2 28 oz. can tomatoes
- ✓ ¼ cup brown rice
- ✓ ½ lb. fresh green beans, cut and/ or 10 oz. package frozen cut green beans
- ✓ 8 oz. can organic kidney beans, undrained or 1 cup home-cooked kidney beans

Directions: In a 6 quart pot, sauté onion, celery, carrots, and garlic until softened. Add stock or water, tomatoes, rice and bay leaf. Bring to a boil and cover, reducing heat to simmer for 50 minutes; stir in kidney beans and green beans and simmer for 5-10 minutes more until all vegetables are tender. Remove bay leaf before serving. Save leftovers for another day.

Calories: 287 Carbs: 53g Protein: 13g Fat: 5g Fiber: 11g

Fruit Salad w/cinnamon

- ✓ 1 orange, peeled and diced
- ✓ 1 apple, diced
- ✓ ½ cup walnuts or pecan, chopped
- ✓ ½ tsp cinnamon

Place the fruit into bowls. Sprinkle with chopped nuts and/or cinnamon.

Calories: 250, Carbs: 43g, Protein: 4g, Fat: 10g, Fiber: 9g

DAY 3

In addition to eliminating foods listed for Days 1 & 2,

✓ ELIMINATE ALL: Gluten grains - wheat, rye, barley, spelt, kamut, and corn.

*NOTE: You may continue to eat rice, tapioca, amaranth, millet, quinoa and buckwheat

PRE-BREAKFAST	Elixir Shot
BREAKFAST	Metabolism Boosting Green Shake **AND** Sweet Squash Smash **OR** Gluten free Oatmeal or Cooked Quinoa Flakes w/ Banana (see Day 1)
SNACK	Detox Green Smoothie
LUNCH	Bean and Spinach Soup
SNACK	Detox Green Smoothie
DINNER	Berry Coconut Smoothie

RECIPES:

Sweet Squash Smash (serves 2)

✓ 1 medium butternut squash, cut into chunks

✓ 2 medium to large sweet potatoes, cut into chunks

✓ ½ tsp ginger

✓ ½ tsp cinnamon Dash of nutmeg

✓ ¼ cup rice (or coconut) milk

Preheat oven to 350 degrees, steam squash and sweet potato until tender. Remove peels and puree in food processor, Add ginger, cinnamon, nutmeg, and rice or coconut milk (add enough to match the consistency of mashed potatoes). Put mixture into 1 ½ quart casserole dish and garnish with a sprinkle of cinnamon. Bake for 15 minutes. (Add 3 tbsps. of Hemp Seeds or Hearts for Added protein). Nutrition info reflects adding hemp seeds.

Calories: 271 Carbs: 46g Protein: 9g Fat: 7g Fiber:9g

Bean and Spinach Soup (serves 3, 368 Calories per serving)

- ✓ 4 cups vegetable broth
- ✓ 2 medium onions, chopped
- ✓ 1 large garlic clove, minced
- ✓ 1 tsp dried oregano
- ✓ Pepper to taste
- ✓ 1-2 cups kidney or red beans
- ✓ 2 cups white kidney beans (cannellini)
- ✓ 1 cup garbanzo beans (chickpeas)
- ✓ 2-3 cups fresh spinach or escarole, washed, drained, and chopped or 10 oz. frozen chopped spinach.

*Note: Beans can be canned (low sodium) or homemade

Combine all ingredients and simmer about 45 minutes, until onions are soft.

Calories: 368, Carbs: 69g, Protein: 21.5g, Fat: 1.5g, Fiber: 17g

DAY 4

In addition to eliminating foods listed for Days 1-3

- ✓ ELIMINATE ALL: - Remaining grains (quinoa, rice, millet, buckwheat) - Nuts and seeds (except sunflower or pumpkin seeds, coconut milk is ok)

- ✓ Note: You now should be eating vegetables, fruits, and legumes only along with your Vegan Protein powder and/or Chicken, turkey, or fresh fish.

- ✓ INCREASE Protein powder mix - 2 scoops twice daily. or 1-2 servings of chicken, fish, turkey (6-8oz for men and 4-6oz for women).

PRE-BREAKFAST	Elixir Shot
BREAKFAST	1-2 Servings of Vegan Protein Shake (w/8oz water) **AND** Gluten free Oatmeal or Cooked Quinoa Flakes w/ Banana or Berries (see Day 1)

SNACK	Metabolism Boosting Green Shake
LUNCH	Spicy Black Beans & Tomatoes (see recipe below), **OR** Mixed Green Salad and veggies of your choice w/Basic Salad Dressing, (see Day 1), **OR** Bean & Spinach Soup (see Day 3)
SNACK	1-2 Servings Vegan Protein Shake (w/water) **OR** Chicken/Fish/Turkey (Men 6-80z, Women 4-6oz)
DINNER	Vegetarian Chili (see recipe below) **OR** Baked Red Potato and Cooked Veggies, **OR** Mixed Green Salad w/Garbanzo Beans and veggies of your choice **OR** a Carrot Salad

RECIPES:

Spicy Black Beans and Tomatoes (serves 2)

- ✓ 1 tsp olive oil
- ✓ 1 small onion, chopped
- ✓ 2 garlic cloves, minced
- ✓ 1 4 oz. can diced green chilies
- ✓ 1/2 tsp cumin
- ✓ 1/2 tsp ground red pepper
- ✓ 1/4 tsp chili powder

- ✓ 1 15 oz. can black beans, drained (low sodium)
- ✓ 1 can chopped stewed tomatoes or 2-3 fresh tomatoes, chopped
- ✓ 1 tbsp. chopped onion and minced garlic in olive oil over medium heat until tender.

Directions: Add tomatoes and green chilies. Reduce heat and cook uncovered for 6-8 minutes or until thickened. Stir in beans and remaining ingredients. Cover and heat 5 minutes more.

Calories: 264, Carbs: 54g, Protein:14g, Fat: 4g, Fiber: 14g

Vegetarian Chili (serves 2)

- ✓ 1 tbsp. olive oil
- ✓ 1 medium onion, chopped
- ✓ 2 whole carrots, diced
- ✓ 4 garlic cloves, minced
- ✓ 1 sweet red bell pepper, chopped
- ✓ 1 green bell pepper, chopped
- ✓ 1 jalapeno pepper, fresh or canned, finely chopped
- ✓ 2 tbsp. chili powder
- ✓ 1 tsp cumin
- ✓ 1 cup cooked kidney beans
- ✓ 1 cup pinto beans
- ✓ 1 28 oz. can tomatoes, chopped (reserve juice)
- ✓ ½ tsp fresh ground pepper
- ✓ 2 tbsp. parsley or cilantro, finely chopped

Directions: In a large, non-aluminum soup kettle, heat oil over low heat; add onion, carrot, garlic, and peppers. Cover and cook until vegetables are very soft, about 10 minutes. Remove lid, add chili powder and cumin and cook an additional 2-3 minutes, stirring occasionally. Add beans tomatoes, and their juice. Simmer 20 minutes. Add pepper. Top bowls of chili with parsley/cilantro.

Calories: 395 Carbs: 66g Protein: 16g Fat: 8g Fiber: 21g

Carrot Salad (serves 1-2)

- ✓ 2 cups carrot, shredded
- ✓ ½ cup celery, diced
- ✓ ¼ cup sunflower seeds
- ✓ 3-4 tbsp. coconut milk
- ✓ 2 tbsp. pineapple juice

Mix all ingredients together and chill for several hours before serving.

Calories: 264 Carbs: 30g Protein: 9g Fat: 13g Fiber:10g

DAY 5

CONTINUE elimination foods listed for Days 1 - 4, as well as legumes (beans, peas, lentils).

✓ EAT ONLY those fruits and vegetables as listed below:

    ✓ Cruciferous vegetables (broccoli, cauliflower, kale, cabbage, Brussels sprouts)

    ✓ Raw greens (red and green lettuce, romaine, spinach, endive, kale)

    ✓ Fresh apples and pears (whole or freshly juiced)

    ✓ Continue with 6-8oz (for men) of Chicken, fish, turkey and 4-6oz (for women) 1-2 times daily; especially if you are NOT doing a vegan protein powder.

    ✓ INCREASE Greens and Vegan Protein Powder

*NOTE: Coconut milk isn't known to cause any allergens according to most research. If you prefer, add water instead to your shake at night.

PRE-BREAKFAST	Elixir Shot
BREAKFAST	Detox Green Smoothie 1-2 Servings of Vegan Protein Powder w/8oz of water
SNACK	Kale Chips
LUNCH	1-2 Servings Vegan Protein Powder w/8oz water **AND** Chicken w/Steamed Veggies (Broccoli, Red kale, and/or Swiss chard) **OR** Chicken w/Oven Roasted Brussel Sprouts w/Apples
SNACK	Detox Green Smoothie
DINNER	Chicken/Turkey/Fish **AND** Mixed Greens, Red Cabbage, and Broccoli Florets **OR** Braised Broccoli
SNACK	1 Apple or Pear

RECIPES:

Kale Chips

- ✓ 1 large head of Kale
- ✓ A small bowl of olive oil
- ✓ Iodized sea salt

Directions: Preheat oven to 425 degrees. Remove kale from stalk, leaving the greens in larger pieces. Place a little olive oil in a bowl, dip your fingers and rub a very light coating of oil over the kale. Lay the kale on a baking sheet and bake for 5 minutes or until it starts to turn a bit brown. Keep an eye on it, it can burn quickly. Turn the kale over and add a little salt, or curry or cumin to taste. Bake with the other side up. Remove and serve. These are a must try!

Calories: 187, Carbs:13g, Protein: 4g, Fat: 15g, Fiber: 3g

Oven Roasted Brussels Sprouts w/Apples (makes 2 servings, 173 calories per serving)

- ✓ 1 pint Brussels sprouts, cleaned and left whole
- ✓ 1 small apple, peeled, cored and cut into eights
- ✓ 1 tsp extra virgin olive oil

Directions: Preheat oven to 375 degrees. In a large bowl, toss Brussels sprouts, apple and oil together. Cover a cookie sheet with aluminum foil; spread apple-Brussels sprouts mixture evenly. Roast uncovered for 20 minutes. Also try with cayenne pepper, lime juice & unsweetened apple juice.

Calories: 173, Carbs: 33g, Protein: 10g, Fat: 3g, Fiber: 12g

Garlic Braised Broccoli (serves 2-3)

- ✓ 1 tbsp. extra virgin olive oil
- ✓ 6 garlic clove, fresh, very finely minced
- ✓ 5 cups 1/2 inch broccoli florets

- ✓ 1/2 tsp sea salt
- ✓ 1/4 cup spring or filtered water

Directions: Place oil and garlic in a skillet over medium-low heat. Cook, stirring frequently, for 2 minutes, but do not burn the garlic. Stir in broccoli, salt and water. Cover and increase heat to high. When you hear a strong sizzle, reduce heat to low and cook for 2-3 minutes, stirring frequently. Serve immediately.

Calories: 150, Carbs: 18g, Protein: 7g, Fat: 8g, Fiber: 6g

DAY 6

- ✓ CONTINUE elimination foods listed for Days 1 - 4, as well as legumes (beans, peas, lentils).

- ✓ Only Eat Fruits and Vegetables listed for Day 5

- ✓ INCREASE Greens and Vegan Protein Powder 1-2 scoops 3 times today (same as Day 5)

PRE-BREAKFAST	Elixir Shot
BREAKFAST	Detox Green Smoothie
	1-2 Servings of Vegan Protein Powder w/8oz of water
SNACK	Detox Green Smoothie
LUNCH	1-2 Servings Vegan Protein Powder w/8oz water w/ a side of Steamed Veggies (Broccoli, Red kale, and/or Swiss chard)
	OR Chicken w/Oven Roasted Brussel Sprouts w/ Apples
SNACK	Detox Green Smoothie
DINNER	1-2 Servings of Vegan protein Powder w/8oz of water **AND**
	Baby spinach & Cauliflower florets topped with Salad Dressing **OR** Garlic-Braised Broccoli
SNACK	1 Apple or Pear

Day 7

- ✓ CONTINUE elimination foods listed for Days 1 - 4, as well as legumes (beans, peas, lentils).

- ✓ Only Eat Fruits and Vegetables listed for Day 5

- ✓ INCREASE Vegan protein powder mix - 1-2 scoops 3-4 times today

PRE-BREAKFAST	Elixir Shot
BREAKFAST	1-2 Servings Vegan Protein Powder w/ 8 oz. of water **AND** 1 whole apple or pear
SNACK	Kale Chips **OR** Detox Green Smoothie
LUNCH	1-2 Servings Vegan protein powder mixed w/8 oz. water **AND** steamed broccoli, red kale, and/or Swiss chard (thinly chopped) topped with olive or flaxseed oil
SNACK	Detox Green Smoothie **OR** Kale Chips
DINNER	1-2 Servings Vegan Protein Powder w/ 8 oz. of water w/mixed greens, red cabbage, and broccoli florets topped with Salad Dressing
SNACK	1-2 Servings Vegan Protein Powder w/8oz water **OR** 1 apple/pear

DAY 8

- ✓ Gently ADD back fruits, vegetables to your diet

PRE-BREAKFAST	Elixir Shot
BREAKFAST	1-2 Servings of Vegan Protein Powder w/water **AND** Banana & Berries w/cinnamon **OR** Tropical Salad **OR** Metabolic Boosting Green Shake
SNACK	Metabolic Boosting Green Shake w/Vegan Protein Powder

LUNCH	Sweet Squash Smash AND Mixed Greens Salad w/ veggies of your choice w/Basic Salad Dressing.
SNACK	Detox Green Smoothie
DINNER	Oven Roasted Veggies **OR** Berry Coconut Smoothie

DAY 9

✓ ADD back: White rice, Quinoa, millet, buckwheat, nuts, seeds and legumes

PRE-BREAKFAST	Elixir Shot
BREAKFAST	1 Serving of Vegan Protein Powder w/8oz of water Oatmeal w/Coconut Milk and Mashed Banana/Berries **OR** Applesauce w/cinnamon and chopped nuts
SNACK	1-2 servings Vegan Protein Powder w/8oz of water **OR** Nuts/Seeds (1-2 Handfuls)
LUNCH	Spicy Black Beans and Tomatoes **OR** Bean & Spinach Soup, **OR** hummus with sliced avocado and tomato on rice cakes (added chicken, turkey, fish if needed).
SNACK	Apple w/Almond Butter, mixed raw nuts, **OR** Protein Shake
DINNER	Vegetarian Chili **OR** Quinoa Salad, **OR** mixed green salad with sliced red bell peppers, red cabbage, garbanzo beans, and sliced onion tossed with Basic Salad Dressing **OR** Berry Coconut Smoothie

Day 10

Congratulations, you have successfully made it to day 10 of the Remodel Detox!

✓ Use your knowledge from this detox and reference Day 9 to create a meal plan for today.

✓ What to do after Day 10: For maximum benefits from this program, it is important to slowly reintroduce the foods which you have not added back to your diet yet. If you suspect that you have food allergies, try only one new food at a time and wait 24 - 48 hours to see if you note a reaction. If unsure about a reaction, wait until symptoms recede and eat only foods that do not cause a reaction. Then ingest the suspicious food again and take note. If you want a complete meal plan visit thelifestylerenovation.com.

THE FRAMEWORK: EXERCISE

Where Do I Start?

'I want to exercise! I want to run, go to the gym, go for a swim, but where do I start?' The hardest part of working out is the anticipation of the actual workout; once you get your butt up, go to the gym, run, swim, or whatever mode you choose you will feel much better! When you work out without a real plan, it's easy to become lost and get discouraged. You may be on a run and not know how far you have gone, you go to the gym but wander around looking at the weights; hoping they will lift themselves (if only it were that easy). Think of it as someone starting a business without a business plan, they will aimlessly be wandering around without a true purpose and hope they make millions. You need to have a clear plan for your workouts. Without a clear path you can't and won't achieve optimal results. Once the clearing exercise has been complete (beginning of the book if you are skipping around) I'm sure you will be raring to go but you need to grab that big ass bull by the horns and create a plan of attack!

185) DO YOUR HOMEWORK!

Think to yourself, when was the last time you had a great workout? Do you know your current fitness levels? If not, I would highly suggest your first workout be a 'getting to know yourself' session where you can find out the answers to fitness questions. These can be: What kind of cardiovascular stamina do I have? What is the heaviest weight I can lift 15 times CONSISTENTLY with GOOD FORM (guys you know what I'm talking about throwing those 100 pound dumbbells around like a scene out of Gladiator; put that down and use the lighter weights before you hurt yourself!)? How many push-ups can I do? All of these questions require answers in order for you to create an exercise plan. Why not run some tests and find these out? It is important when lifting weights, you can complete several sets of each exercise with proper form; otherwise there is no point. Have you ever seen the person in the gym that goes from machine to machine, does a few reps on each and then leaves like they did something? This is pretty much useless and won't require enough of a muscular stimulus for your body to adapt and change for the better; you might as well sit your ass on the couch! You may be able to lift a dumbbell for one repetition, but that doesn't mean you should start with that weight. Find a weight (or bodyweight exercise) that you are comfortable with and perform 10-15 reps with GOOD FORM and do this for several sets of each exercise. Your muscles need to develop endurance just like you have to develop cardiovascular endurance to run a consistent distance time and time again. Once you are comfortable with resistance training then you can start picking up big boy or big girl weights with proper form and hone in on your fitness goals even more! Don't set the bar too high for yourself for the first few workouts, literally; Rome wasn't built in a day and neither will your ideal birthday suit!

186) DEVELOP YOUR PLAN OF ACTION!

Once you know what kind of shape you are in, you can then begin to plan a fitness program. Now that you know what to include and what areas you need to work on in terms of strength, endurance and conditioning, you can develop a plan. When creating your workout plan, first you have to decide when and for how long you will be available. Try to set a certain time aside each day. For example, if you get home from work at six o'clock in the evening, you could leave 7-8 as your 'workout time' (45 minutes to an hour is sufficient). At first, you can build a program that works the full body (all muscle groups) for time and efficiency to complete three times a week; one exercise for each muscle group. EASY, RIGHT? Be sure to vary your exercises to keep it fresh and keep challenging yourself. Once you begin to feel comfortable, you can create a workout specific to muscle groups into separate workout days. For example, you could work biceps and triceps on one day, back and shoulders the next and so on. Don't worry; I'll help you get started with exercise ideas and workout plans found later in this chapter.

187) DEAR DIARY...OR FITNESS APP!

When working out, it can be helpful to keep a diary or journal so that you can keep track of everything you have done. It can be extremely motivating to see all of your workouts written down in front of you! You can also compare performances from a previous workout; you can say 'Oh yeah! I ran that same distance but I shaved two minutes off of the time!' There are also many fitness apps that can help you organize and keep track of this information.

188) GET CREATIVE...NOT FANCY!

Next, if you can invest in some equipment then go ahead (if you will use it for more than a coat rack); but if not, DO NOT WORRY! I hear this excuse far too often...I can't afford it. Just because you can't afford a gym membership or fancy fitness equipment doesn't mean you can't get a good workout in! It is an excuse that I hear FAR too often and I will not accept it because excuses are like buttholes, everyone has one and they are surely full of s%@*!! With a simple pair of athletic shoes you have several effective exercises available to you like running, walking (yes you can do the mall walk like the cute old ladies), hiking, jumping rope, bodyweight exercises, and more! Take a look around you right now, what do you see? There are MANY exercises that can be done just on the floor (or on the back of your couch), so I GUARANTEE you can find something around your house to use as a makeshift weight (jugs of water, cans of beans, candle sticks, even a towel can be used to break a sweat (not just wipe it off)! I'm not saying that this is the most efficient way of training, but a bit of creativity can go a long way and make do until you have saved enough money to buy a set of dumbbells or bands!

189) LISTEN TO YOUR BODY!

Finally, when working out (especially in the first few weeks) it is important to listen to what your body is telling you. A lot of people, and I mean A LOT of people, that experience pain after workouts think because they are 'new' to certain exercises or because they are 'using muscles that they haven't used in a long time,' it is nothing of concern. Although this is partly true, any serious pain that doesn't get better after a few days, should be seen by a doctor as you may have a bigger underlying problem. Just don't use a little muscle soreness as an excuse to quit!

When Is The Best Time To Work Out?

190) MORNING VS. AFTERNOON WORKOUTS!

I get asked this question a lot by people and the best answer I can give them is to work out when you will make it a habit! Whether you work out in the morning, mid-day, or afternoon, just get moving and make it a habit! If you are a man you could slightly benefit from a morning workout as your testosterone levels are highest in the morning around 9am (hence morning wood) making it possible to lift more weight. At the end of the day, it all comes down to your personal preference. Some of us are early risers and if you can consistently exercise before work, that's great. If rising early makes you cringe, and the thought of leaving your cozy bed to go to the gym is unbearable, try a workout during lunch time for an energy boost or a session after work to release the stressors of your day! In the end the best option for you is the one that will motivate you to work out.

✓ **Benefits of exercising in the morning** – People who exercise before work in general tend to stick to their plan a bit better. They have gotten it out of the way before other time constraints effect their day. It is much easier to find an excuse to skip an evening exercise session than a morning one. The ONLY excuse you have to skip a morning workout is because you want to stay in bed longer! Try to set your alarm and place it away from you so you have to physically get out of bed to turn it off; this way you are less likely to hit snooze!

✓ **Benefits of exercising later in the day** – On the other hand, some people find that they do not feel the full benefit of a morning workout because they are still half asleep! You may find it better to let your body get into the swing of the day before you exercise.

It is all down to personal preference! The important thing to remember is to find what is comfortable for YOU and only you. Why not try a week of morning workouts and then a week of evening workouts and see how your body adjusts to the different time schedules? As long as you choose a time of day that can be repeated on a daily basis then you will find yourself exercising consistently in no time!

Before A Workout

191) DO: SET A GOAL!

Set a goal to work out an hour a day…it doesn't even have to be all at once! If you set a goal to work out for an hour a day this doesn't mean it has to be consecutive! Work out 3 times in a day for 20 minutes each or two half hours sessions. Working out multiple times a day for shorter amounts of time will keep your metabolism up and allow your food to be used as energy. Get up in the morning and go for a run or do 20 minutes of stretching, go for a walk during lunch, and get a quick session in the gym after work, boom!!! An hour! Take away all of your crap excuses about not having time to fit an hour workout in since now you know that it doesn't have to be all at once!

192) DO: PREPARE YOURSELF!

By this, I mean take a look at your plan for today and get into your head EXACTLY what you will be doing! Commit it to memory or write it down! This will make your daily goal clear, set the standard and allow the workout to flow in a smooth manner!

193) DO: EAT FOR FUEL!

This tip can provide you with extra energy when it finally comes time to work out. About an hour before, you want to consume a food or drink that will give you energy DURING the workout; something that will help you to run that extra minute, or push out three more reps on the weights. A nut butter on toast is a good option as it will give you carbs, fat AND protein! A good protein shake or bar will also do the trick!

194) DO: CARB UP TO PUMP UP!

When you resistance train with bodyweight, weights, bands, or perform high intensity exercise your body uses carbs for energy. Your muscles rely on carbs stored in your muscles. The body is also able to use carbs that are still in the blood from a meal earlier in the day. The meal before your training should include slow-digesting carbs or a combination of slow- and medium-acting carbs. Slow-burning carbs will prevent you from crashing during training (and possibly dropping a weight on your pretty face), and the body can use some of the carbs for fuel as muscle glycogen stores become depleted during the workout. Carbs which digest somewhat faster include bananas, potatoes, pasta, apples, oranges, coconut oil/flakes, and brown rice. These will be even more readily available for the body to draw on. About 30 minutes to an hour before your weight training workout have 20-40 grams of low glycemic carbs with about 20 grams of whey protein.

*Note: If your goal is to lose body fat and you will be performing cardio only do NOT eat a lot of carbs beforehand; a little protein is best (about 20 grams) to prevent muscle breakdown; unless you are training fasted (refer to hack #48).

195) DO: TAKE YOUR SUPPLEMENTS!

Whether it is the supplements that I have suggested previously or a different choice, make sure you take your supplements about a half an hour before you intend to work out. Most contain caffeine and amino acids that will help increase your blood flow via dilated veins and arteries!

196) DO: TAKE YOUR BCAAs!

BCAAs or Branched Chain Amino Acids should be an important part of your workouts. BCAAs are the building blocks of protein! There are three BCAAs; Valine, Leucine and Isoleucine. Leucine is the most researched and appears to offer the most benefits. BCAAs provide the basis for 'protein synthesis' and the production of energy which is vital when you want to work out! BCAAs are rare in that they head straight for the bloodstream and are not degraded by the liver. Consuming BCAAs before a workout can increase uptake into muscle tissue, which is what we all want, right? It can also increase growth hormone and muscular oxidization. BCAAs are also great before cardio in the morning on an empty stomach as they will prevent your body from using muscle as energy and instead utilize more fat as energy, nice! Try adding 5-10 grams to your pre and post-workout routine! (Note if you are lifting high volume you may want to consider adding some BCAAs to your water and sip while you work out to provide your muscles with constant energy).

197) DO: PROTEIN AND CREATINE!

You may have heard A LOT of talk about which supplements are the best to avoid and best to take! TAKE PROTEIN AND CREATINE if you want to build muscle! It is thought that people who consumed these two BEFORE AND AFTER THEIR WORKOUTS showed a significant boost in muscle growth (and bench press strength) compared to those who didn't. It is also important to take protein and creatine before and after workouts as opposed to before bed and early morning as the differences can be astounding!

198) DO: COFFEE BEFORE WORKOUT!

Research has shown that consuming coffee a couple of hours before your workout can bring some great benefits! It can reduce the pain and strain that your muscles feel during the workout meaning that you can complete more reps as well as increasing the amount of fat you can burn! One cup generally does the trick. If coffee isn't to your liking feel free to substitute with a caffeinated tea. Just remember caffeine is a stimulant and too much can cause ill effects.

199) DO: DRINK PLENTY OF WATER!

The recommended amount of water before exercise is 20 ounces; we don't want to go too overboard as we will end up losing more than we retain through constant toilet breaks. Water will help to keep us hydrated and can prevent dizziness and muscle cramping; we also tend to perform better during the workout when sufficiently hydrated!

200) DO: WARM UP!

You walk into the gym, raring to go and jump straight into your workout! NO, NO, NO! You HAVE to warm up before a workout! This is vital as it will help to get the blood pumping around your body. You will also be stretching your muscles in order to prevent strain and possible injury when you get started. Sometimes you may go to the gym with others and they may head STRAIGHT into a workout and you feel a little strange warming up first, DON'T! In fact, make it a habit to warm up together. A warmup can be several things like a slow jog, riding a bike, running in place, or doing some bodyweight or light weight exercises, such as squats, pushups, or walking lunges to get your body prepared (DO NOT lift heavy your first set before your muscles are warm).

201) DO NOT: STRETCH COLD!

Contrary to popular belief stretching before your muscles and tissues are warm can lead to injury. What you want to do is warm up to get your blood flowing first and then stretch if you desire. Just remember, although you should feel slight tension during a stretch, it should never be painful.

202) DO NOT: OVERSLEEP!

You have just got home from work and you have over an hour before you are heading off to the gym so you decide get in a quick power-nap for 15-20 minutes. This can be great as you will wake up feeling refreshed and ready to go. However, if you sleep any more than 30 minutes, this will have the opposite effect and you will actually feel more tired. Napping before a workout longer than 30 minutes will make it difficult to get up, easier to press the snooze button, and next thing you know you haven't gone to the gym, you have missed dinner and you have woken up shortly before you were planning to go to sleep tonight! ABSOLUTE DISASTER!

203) DO NOT: OVERDO THE SUPPLEMENTS!

While a dose of caffeine and amino acids will leave you feeling pumped and full of energy, too much will tip this over the edge and leave you with a rapid heart rate, anxiety, and a general feeling of illness which will severely affect your workout! NEVER take more than a recommended dose unless you are instructed by your health care professional.

204) DO NOT: STRESS!

'Stress is the cause of all disease'. When you stress, you tend to release cortisol which breaks down muscle tissue and encourages the storage of fat! Stress will also prevent you from being able to focus and concentrate during a workout and will ultimately leave you feeling frustrated!

205) DO NOT: PERFORM HIGH INTENSITY CARDIO BEFORE WEIGHTS!

Performing 'steady state' cardio before weights can be really effective as your body is burning fat and you still have the ability to lift and complete your sets. However, 'high intensity' cardio will have the opposite effect and it will interfere with your anaerobic process as well as reduce your power when lifting!

206) DO NOT: EAT TOO MUCH!

As I have said, a pre workout snack can be highly beneficial, but eating too much will lead to stomach cramps and a general 'uncomfortable feeling' during the work-out. It will also reduce the effectiveness of your exercise because more blood will be focused on digesting the food rather than flow to your muscles! Believe me I have had countless clients blow chunks when working out because their food hasn't had time to digest, gross!

207) DO NOT: HAVE REFINED CARBS BEFORE A WORKOUT!

I hear this ALL OF THE TIME from people, 'well I'm going to work out so I can have something sweet since I'm going to 'burn it off anyway!' This simply is NOT a good idea! Avoid refined carbs such as candy, fat free muffins, and processed sugars (refer to hack #45).Yes, these carbs burn rapidly, but they burn so fast that eventually you will run on fumes. This can short circuit your energy, causing blood sugar levels to surge (limiting fat burning) and then drastically drop, which will make you feel weak. For example, have you ever seen a little kid's sports game and witness kids eating processed crap before a game or during half time and you wonder why some of them seem to simply run out of energy? Yup, bingo, this is why! Giving kids sugar because they are 'skinny' or they will 'work it off' is like saying, 'they have healthy lungs so they can have a cigarette!' Don't do it!

After A Workout

Many people finish their workout and then are done for the day; they don't consider the things that they should do once they have finished. Luckily for you, I am here to give you some great tips to maximize the effectiveness of your hard work (as well as some things that you should NEVER do)!

208) DO: COOL DOWN!

Don't make a hasty exit as soon as you finish your last set, doing some light cardio can help to remove any metabolic waste! Try to target the area that you have just worked out so you are keeping it relevant. For example, if you have just worked out your upper body, hop on the rowing machine for a few minutes!

209) DO: STRETCH!

Stretching can be REALLY important after a workout as it helps the nervous system relax and recover along with the muscles. A good stretch should feel slightly uncomfortable but NEVER painful! If you overstretch, you are likely to cause an injury even after your muscles are warmed up!

210) DO: ROLL!

I cannot emphasize the importance of this tip enough! You have to prepare yourself because this WILL hurt, especially after an intense workout. Using a foam roller before your stretch will help to improve flexibility, circulation and most importantly, break up knots that may appear in your soft tissue. This can also be done as a warm-up exercise before you work out!

211) DO: REHYDRATE!

If you have just pushed your body to the limit and you are sweating, it means you have lost water from your body, make sure you replenish this after a workout. Proper hydration will lubricate the joints as well as regulate your body temperature!

212) DO: AFTER RESISTANCE TRAINING CONSUME PROTEIN!

In several studies subjects who consumed protein and carbohydrates within 1-2 hours (known as the 'Anabolic Window') of resistance training added more muscle than those who waited more than 2 hours [30]. After a workout, your body needs to replace all the nutrients that have been lost, such as amino acids and carbs! Your body needs these to repair the muscle cells and feed the nervous system. So make sure that you include around 20 grams of protein (and up to 50 for athletes and people who train hard) to encourage protein synthesis, aka muscle recovery! Whey protein is a great option because it is digested quickly and provides our muscle cells with much-needed amino acids. When the goal is more muscle, you cannot afford to lose your whey!

213) DO: AFTER RESISTANCE TRAINING CONSUME SIMPLE CARBS!

If you are lifting weights and doing resistance training, carbs need to be taken in to help aid the recovery of your muscle, joints, and tissues. This is the ONE time when you want to consume a HIGH CARB and high glycemic food, nice! A great option is a potassium rich food like a banana, coconut water, or white potato coupled with a protein shake (see hack above). These are great because your potassium reserves will inevitably be shot from an intense workout session. Potassium, among other nutrients like calcium and sodium are key minerals which play a role in muscular energy. You may also opt for some white rice with some protein powder mixed in it (add water or cashew milk) to create a delicious rice protein pudding. You can even have some white bread with a protein shake or a sandwich with lean protein. One thing you do NOT want to do though is have a lot of fiber or fat post weight training as this will limit the insulin spike; which we WANT after a weight training session to help deliver nutrients into the muscle. An insulin spike is NOT necessary post weight training but it will be helpful for you muscle recovery, growth, and repair.

Now if you are really looking to indulge (NOT RECOMMENDED) this is the BEST TIME to do so! I tell people to get a good percentage of their daily carbs post resistance training; about 30% so they can replenish their muscles and avoid fat gain. *Do NOT do this post cardio session as you don't want to spike your insulin level as this will halt any fat burning effort by your body.

214) DO: WEAR TIGHT CLOTHING!

Compression clothing is easy to find nowadays and has been shown to benefit your workout as well as help you recover AFTER your workout! Compression clothing will help get more oxygenated blood into the muscles, remove metabolic waste, and aid in recovery. (Plus they keep everything tight and in place, making you look hot, hot, hot!)

215) DO: TAKE ANTI-INFLAMMATORIES!

According to some studies, anti-inflammatory medications and spices such as turmeric and ginger can speed muscle recovery and reduce inflammation [19]. Important note: if you are trying to build muscle, NSAIDs (drugs like ibuprofen and aspirin), may hinder hypertrophy (muscle growth). In other words, if you want bigger chesticles (pecs) or any other muscle NSAIDs could inhibit that [20]!

216) DO: TAKE BCAAS AND GLUTAMINE!

Most protein powders have your essential branched chain amino acids within the powder which include leucine, isoleucine, and valine. The essential amino acids (not made by the body) can help aid in your workout (as discussed earlier) and help you recover, grow, and maintain muscle tissue. Along with BCAAs another great option to add is the most abundant amino acid in the body, Glutamine. Glutamine has been shown to increase growth hormone levels, boost your immune system, repair a leaky gut for proper gut health, cure ulcers, preserve muscle tissue and help increase protein synthesis to repair and build muscle. In a study by the American College of Sports Medicine (ACSM), Glutamine taken before a workout has been shown to increase muscular output and energy. Subjects lost no strength during glutamine supplementation versus the placebo group and were also able to train longer and harder without any loss in muscular output. How to use these two supplements? If your protein powder has BCAAs and glutamine in it simply drink a shake before and after your workout. Otherwise on training days, consume 20-50 grams of BCAAS and 5-10g of Glutamine before and after your workout. On non-training days consume 20-50 of BCAAs and 5-10 grams of glutamine throughout the day.

217) DO: TAKE CREATINE TO ADD MUSCLE!

Creatine after a workout helps you get bigger and stronger; research has shown that post-workout creatine consumption is more effective than pre-workout consumption [31].

218) DO: TAKE VITAMIN D!

Vitamin D should be taken daily as it helps decrease inflammation, fight obesity, prevent arthritis, protect against radiation, improve your immune system, give you stronger bones, prevent cancer, help with brain health, reduce risk of heart disease, and has been shown to magnify the muscle building effects of leucine (an amino acid) [32]. Take 2,000 IU's a day, 1,000 IU's in the morning and 1,000 IU's after a workout is a good regiment (some healthcare professionals recommend 5,000 IU's of vitamin D at a time). Simply check with your healthcare provider if you have questions.

219) DO NOT: TAKE 2 DAYS OFF IN A ROW!

Not working out for two days in a row can slow your metabolic rate slightly, and we want to keep it up as long as possible! Instead of working out for 5 or 6 days straight and then taking two days of complete rest, train 3 or 4 days and then take a day off, followed by another 3 – 4 days of training.

220) DO NOT: DO TOO MUCH CARDIO!

As I have said, a short session of cardio after a weight session can be beneficial but too much will have the opposite effect. You can end up damaging the hormonal mechanisms that lead to muscular hypertrophy (growth). Cardio after weights can help burn fat; just don't train for your marathon afterwards! 20-30 minutes of low intensity cardio is a good choice like walking on the treadmill or a slow bike ride.

221) DO NOT: LAY AROUND THE NEXT DAY!

I hear this ALL OF THE TIME from people complaining that they are too sore from the workout the day before to actually do any activity; 'Joey, I can't even sit down go to the bathroom because I'm so sore!' Look, you shouldn't be so debilitated from your workout that you can't walk the next day, but if you are you need to MOVE!!! When you complete some light cardio, stretch, and/or foam roll, it gets blood flowing to your tissues (especially the sore ones) and will help relieve your muscle soreness and repair your tissue faster. Think of this like a necessary massage to work on the muscle tissue and bring blood into the area.

222) DO NOT: SKIP RESTING TIME!

The perfect scenario would include your workout followed by a short nap; realistically speaking we know that is unlikely. When possible, try to relax and not do anything too strenuous in the hours after your workout to allow your body to recover faster!

Every Day Exercises

Stay healthy every day with these **6 Exercises. Spending 6 minutes** a day to help limit injury and help you move and feel better!

223) COBRA PUSH-UP!

Lower back pain affects 60-80% of the population and there IS, yes, there IS a way to avoid going under the knife! We need to make sure we have strong glutes, lower back, hips, groin, and abs. Strengthening these muscles and staying loose will alleviate tension on your back. Try the cobra push-up every morning or whenever you feel stiffness in your back. This is mainly a stretching exercise and stretches the lower back, groin, abs, and hip flexors.

- ✓ **Here's how to Cobra:** Lay down on the floor with your chest, stomach, and thighs flat to the ground. Place your palms flat on the ground and in line with your arm pits, elbows bent. Keep your chin tucked in (double chin might happen). Your goal is to keep the lower half of your body on the ground (imagine your hips glued to the floor), but always keeping your butt and lower back relaxed. Just using your arm strength (do not squeeze your butt or tense your back) push upwards so your upper body lifts off the ground keeping your hips, pelvis, and quads on the floor. Once you reach the top exhale through your mouth to release any tightness in your back. Hold for 5 seconds and then lower yourself back down to the ground. Complete at least 10 times.

224) TUSHY SQUEEZE!

We are living in a time where everyone (well, mostly everyone) wants to have a nice thick booty. But (pun intended) we have an epidemic of people with weak glutes. If your butt is not firing (activating) while working out (or even walking for that matter) this can be the root of your back pain. Your glutes need to work correctly to take the load off of your lower back. Fix that by squeezing your butt 30 seconds a day! Doing this can get your glutes to fire properly, take away pain from your lower back, and get your butt ready for a leg intensive work out!

✓ **Here's how:** simply stand with your feet shoulder width apart, feet turned out slightly. Now squeeze your butt like you are trying to hold a quarter between your cheeks. At the same time squeeze your abs and tighten your fists as hard as you can. Squeezing all of these simultaneously will give a better muscular contraction known as muscular irradiation. Hold the squeeze for 30 seconds (believe me this is hard), remember to breathe, and after all is said and done you will have a higher neuromuscular capacity, limit injury to your spine, and quite possibly have a better tushy!

225) DEEP SQUAT!

Many people have hip flexion and mobility issues. Doing a deep bodyweight squat will truly help you with your hip mobility. This practice is done in many Asian and Middle Eastern countries and requires 90-130 degrees of hip flexion (your hip bend) and 110-165 degrees of knee flexion (how much your knees bend). Doing this will help prevent possible hip replacements when you are older and also allow you to have better form and strength when lifting.

✓ **Here's how:** Do NOT load any weight with this exercise; especially on your back. This exercise is performed simply to retain and encourage hip and knee mobility. Squat down as low as you can with your feet flat on the ground not letting your heels come up. It IS OK to let your back round out at the bottom of this motion as you do not have any weight loaded on your back. Squat as low as you can where your butt almost touches the ground (the more you do these the more mobility you will gain), hold for 30 seconds and slowly rise up, just once is all you need every day!

226) HAMSTRING STRETCH!

When our hamstrings get tight it can lead to a number of problems like a tight back and glutes, possible injuries when lifting, and plantar fasciitis (pain in the bottom of the foot). If your hamstrings are tight you will compensate and use your lower back to lift anything and possibly risk throwing your back out or worse. The saying 'lift with your legs' still holds true!

✓ **How:** Sit down with your feet outstretched and try to bend forward to touch your toes (or as close as you can). You can also stand up and bend over for a good stretch. Hold for 30 seconds for each leg and do this once a day at a minimum!

227) 'T' STRETCH / WALL STRETCH!

As a sedentary society, our posture increasingly worsens the more we stay put. This contributes to a host of problems such as tight neck, sore shoulders, weak pecs, and lower back pain, to name a few. We can help alleviate these issues by doing a simple stretch, called the T-stretch every day to lengthen our tight shoulders, chest, and forward head position.

✓ **Here's how:** Stand tall and extend your arms outward in a T position while sticking your chest out and externally rotating your shoulders so that your thumbs are behind you. Bring your hands back so that your shoulders blades squeeze together. Keep your head in a neutral position by tucking your chin down (hello double chin again), hold the position for 3-5 seconds and repeat 10 times. This can also be done between a door frame extending your arms out, one palm on each side of the door frame and walk forward so that you feel a stretch in your shoulders and chest. Hold for 30 seconds.

228) DIAPHRAGM BREATHING!

The simple act of breathing deeply can be incredibly beneficial. It can lower our stress levels, lower our heart rate, and can balance our nervous system. Learning how to breathe from your diaphragm can make a world of difference.

✓ **Here's how:** Lie down on your back (great thing to do when you first wake up in the morning). Place one hand on your chest and one hand on top of your belly button. Simply take a deep breath; taking notice to breathe in through your nose so that your belly raises first (bringing air into your stomach) and the last third of the inhalation is where you will see your chest rise. Exhale through your mouth about twice as long as the inhalation. Do this for 4-5 minutes every day!

Efficient and Effective Exercises

Look, I get it, we are living in an increasingly busy world and we barely have time to answer an email let alone find time to exercise. This is exactly why we need to be as efficient as possible and make the most out of our workouts! I have compiled a list of the most EFFICIENT and EFFECTIVE exercises to save you from wasting time when push comes to shove and you need to get in a workout in a short amount of time!

Hey ladies, this is for you as well! Many women skip past the weights because they don't want to become 'muscular' when the truth is, women DO NOT have enough testosterone to put on muscle like men. Women will benefit from weight lifting tremendously! Ladies, if you truly want to have tight abs, arms that don't flap in the wind, and a tight lifted booty then you HAVE to lift weights and resistance train! Simply doing cardio may get you to lose weight but it WON"T change your frame, muscle density, or make your skin tighter! Resistance training can boost your metabolism and help you burn fat. In fact, cardio and resistance training complement each other very well; as the cardio and weight lifting will help you to lose weight and lifting will also help to tighten the skin. You can also lower blood pressure, reduce the risk of heart problems and diabetes as muscles help to remove glucose from the bloodstream!

NOTE: For demonstrations of ALL exercises listed please visit my YouTube page: www.youtube.com/c/joeythurmanfit.

229) PEE ON THE HYDRANT!

You want me to what?! This is one of my favorite exercises (the name helps) because it causes a great deal of muscular stability, core engagement (especially those pesky obliques), and can really get your heart rate elevated to burn some fat!

- ✓ **HOW?** Get on your hands in a pushup position. Lift one leg slightly in the air while keeping your abs tight, a flat back, and shoulders engaged. Take the leg that is in the air and pull your knee towards the elbow on the same side (right knee to right elbow). Try to bring you knee as far as you can towards your arm so that your knee is as close to your elbow as possible. Squeeze your abs and pause (yes, the image of a dog using a fire hydrant might come to mind) then extend the leg back out and repeat for 10-20 on each side!

230) THE DEADLIFT!

The beast that is the deadlift! 'Why is this exercise so great for your body?' Because it targets SO MANY muscles! It is a true whole body movement since it engages your torso, back, legs, abs, hamstrings and more! As a result, we release a HUGE amount of muscle-building testosterone into the bloodstream as well as increase fat burning, elevate growth hormone, and elevate metabolism. This is a great exercise for lower back health and for developing a nice set of glutes (booty). This move will also make your hamstrings flexible which means that you are less likely to get back pain after sitting all day (this is EXTREMELY useful if you have an office job and are stuck in a chair). For this reason, the deadlift should be one of your MAIN priorities when working out! *Note: if you have lower back problems start with a very light weight doing this exercises or if you aren't comfortable you can use a hamstring curl machine or perform a hamstring curl using a ball lying on your back.

✓ **HOW?** Start by standing upright with a dumbbell in each hand with your palm facing towards you (you may also use an alternating grip with one hand facing you and one hand facing outward). Keeping your arms straight and your knees slightly bent, slowly bend at your hips and lower the weights as far as you can without changing the shape of your back, which should remain straight. Now squeeze your glutes to pull yourself back up. It is important to bend at the hips (rather than the waist) and pull yourself up with your glutes (rather than your back). *Note, this movement allows for more mobility if you use dumbbells; you can use a barbell when you get more comfortable.

231) THE SQUAT!

Just like the deadlift, the barbell back squat also hits most of the major muscle groups and is one of the best exercises for developing your legs! When athletes were asked how they could run so fast, jump so high and have all over improved strength, squats were the answer. This can be done with a barbell on your back, dumbbells to your side or without weights at all.

✓ **HOW?** Start by getting under the barbell in the rack, dipping your head underneath it and rest it onto your upper back. Next, bring your feet in underneath you, shoulder width apart. When you feel ready, un-rack the bar by straightening your legs and begin to squat remembering to keep your lower back neutral. You have to BREAK parallel; getting your thighs parallel to the floor IS NOT enough! You have to dip your hips BELOW your knees. Squat back up keeping your chest up, abs tight, and locking your hips and knees into place; and don't forget to breathe!

232) THE PULL-UP!

The pull-up is easy and doesn't require much space or equipment and the results can be phenomenal! Daily pull-ups will lead to sculpted shoulders and lats! It is also a big multi-joint movement which will allow for an increase in testosterone release leading to bigger and better muscle strength!

✓ **HOW?** Grab the pullup handles with outstretched arms and pull your body up as far as possible by drawing your shoulder blades together with your "lats." Your back should remain straight and your arm muscles should not be used any more than necessary. Remember to keep abs tight. Lower yourself slowly until your arms are almost fully extended. May be done on an assisted pullup machine or swapped out for a lat pulldown as well.

233) THE PUSH-UP!

Push-ups are by far one of the most underrated exercises around! Push-ups not only work your chest muscles but they involve core stability, shoulder strength and stability, work the muscles of your back, work on body awareness, and work your triceps. The great thing about pushups is you don't need any equipment except your own bodyweight and ingenuity! These can be done on the ground, on your knees, on a bench, on the back of your couch, against the wall, with your feet in straps, feet elevated, on a ball, or any combination you can think of.

✓ **HOW?** Place hands farther than shoulder width so your arms can create a 90 degree angle when in a bent position. Keeping legs stiff and core tight, bend the elbows so that your chest is just above the floor. Extend the elbows and repeat. Make sure to lead with the chest, bringing the chest closest to the floor and do not to let the lower back sink. If you are a beginner, keep your knees on the floor.

234) MEDICINE BALL SLAM!

This is a FANTASTIC exercise for carving those abs and mid-drifts. It also contains a level of cardio too so will help to maintain your sculpted abs!

✓ **HOW?** It is super easy and just involves slamming the medicine ball into the floor and catching it (if it bounces) or squatting down (keeping correct form in mind) and picking it back up. Once you have caught the ball, lift it above your head and slam it back down into the floor!

235) THE BENCH PRESS!

Probably the main question people who go to the gym get asked is 'What do you bench?' This is because this exercise demonstrates the strength of your triceps, shoulders and pecs. It is a great exercise for developing a more powerful upper-body and is the one of the most effective for changing your appearance and developing a presence!

✓ **HOW?** Start by lying on the bench with your eyes under the bar. Lift your chest and squeeze your shoulder blades back making sure that your feet are flat on the floor or flat on the bench, keeping your back flat. Grab the bar tightly in the base of your palm keeping your wrists straight. Take a deep breath and un-rack the bar by straightening your arms. Bring the bar above your shoulders keeping your elbows locked. Lower the bar to your chest, tucking your elbows in and then pushing it back up, locking your elbows at the top. Make sure you have someone there to 'spot' you just in case you need help at any point.

236) THE AB CRUNCH WITH A PELVIC TILT!

When done effectively, crunches are one of the best exercises when wanting to strengthen your abdominal muscles. Adding the pelvic tilt allows you to engage the lower muscles region of your abdomen as well. You should try to avoid pulling your neck forward with your hands. You should also avoid holding your breath and always keep your elbows OUT of your line of vision. If you are making any of these mistakes, you could severely be limiting your chances at achieving those desired abs!

✓ **HOW?** Lie flat on the floor, bend your knees and place your hands on the back of your head or across your chest. Flatten your back to the floor and bring your belly button to your spine. Contract your abs and raise your shoulders off of the floor. Slowly breathe out on the way up while keeping your neck straight. As you crunch up drive through your heels to slightly lift your butt off of the ground (tilting your hips towards your chest) to engage your lower abdominal region. Stay at the top for a few seconds then lower yourself back down not fully relaxing at the bottom and repeat!

237) THE BURPEE!

Burpees hurt, we all know they do, but it just means that it is a GREAT exercise for a number of muscles! With every single repetition, you will be working your arms, quads, glutes, chest, abs AND hamstrings! Burpees will help you to rapidly burn fat, boost your metabolism and condition you like CRAZY!

✓ **HOW?** Start by standing with your feet shoulder width apart. The first move is to squat down into an imaginary chair. From here put your hands on the floor and thrust your legs back to put you in the push-up position. Be sure to keep your abs tight and do not let your hips drop down. Keep your arms locked out and frog jump your legs back into the squat position, keeping your chest up and focus forward. Finish off with a burst upwards ending in a small jump off the floor. REPEAT, REPEAT, REPEAT, and feel the burn!

238) THE PLANK!

Planks are one the best exercises you can do to truly work your "core" or in other words your abs, lower back, and trunk stabilizers. Planks will help strengthen your lower back and abs by stabilizing your body and making it more resilient to injury. Planks also give great control to your abs so when you are on the beach you can suck that gut in with the best of them, ha!

✓ **HOW?** Begin in a kneeling position. Place your forearms on the ground so that your elbows are beneath your shoulders and your forearms are parallel to each other (without your hands touching). Extend your legs, locking knees and pointing toes. Elbows should be directly under shoulders. Make sure your lower back does not sink while you hold the plank position. Hold for as long as possible. Lower and repeat. There are no repetitions for this exercise.

The challenge is to simply hold the position. Planks may also be done on your hands or as a side plank to engage more of your oblique's (love handles).

✓ **For a side plank**: Begin by lying on your side with your body in a straight line and one foot on top of the other. The bottom elbow should be bent at 90 degrees and directly below the shoulder. The other arm can be placed on the hip. Using your core, lift your body up off of the floor pushing your hips towards the ceiling and hold for the longest time possible (a good time is 30 seconds or more). Lower and repeat on the other side.

239) THE ROW!

A dumbbell or machine rowing motion is a necessity when working out. The row involves using the muscle of your back to allow for better posture to help take pressure off of the lower back and spine; a major issue for people experiencing back pain. The row uses the muscles of the back (lats, rhomboids, traps, and more), works on stabilizing your core, involves the biceps, and uses the posterior (back) part of your shoulders to round your frame out nicely

✓ *HOW?* **Dumbbell Row**: With one leg, kneel on a bench (stool or chair) for stability, with the other leg extended to the floor. Right arm is extended on top of bench for stability. Left arm is extended at your side hanging with dumbbell in hand. Left palm should be facing in. With a flat back pull the left elbow bringing the dumbbell to your waist. Pull the elbow as far past your back as you can and squeeze your back. Lower the weight and repeat. When you are finished with your repetitions repeat on the other side switching legs and arms to opposite positions.

✓ *HOW?* **Machine Row**: In a seated position bend the knees slightly. Make sure back is straight and arms should be extended grasping handles with palms facing in. Pull the handle into the chest puffing out the chest as you pull. Slide elbows past your back squeezing your rhomboids together (think of crushing a can between your shoulders), hold for a second, return arms to an extended position and repeat. *When doing this exercise make sure to keep your back flat and abs engaged to take pressure off of the lower back.

How Many Reps And Sets Should I Complete?

REPS: First of all, you have to ask yourself whether you are looking to achieve muscle strength or muscle endurance. This will have a direct impact on how many repetitions you will complete with each set. To realize this, you have to know what each 'rep range' will do for your body. If you are looking to gain as much strength as possible you need to pick a heavy weight, so if the weight isn't heavy enough to tax your muscular system you won't achieve your desired results. If you simply complete 1-5 reps with a light weight you will not experience maximal strength gains. Muscle strength and development can only be achieved by using a weight where it is hard to complete more reps than the intended rep range. *Note: The weight, tempo, and form that you use are just as important as the selected rep range.

- ✓ **1-5 reps** – This is mainly used to achieve maximum strength gains. The weight that you use in an exercise with this amount of reps will be high and you will need to make sure that your form is on point! You cannot afford poor form when using a heavy weight.

- ✓ **6-8 reps** – This is a nice middle ground between muscular gains and developing strength. Thus a good range to stay in if you are looking to get stronger with some muscle development.

- ✓ **8-12 reps** – This is the range where you will see the most muscle development (hypertrophy). To see maximum growth you should pick a weight that doesn't allow you to do more than 12 reps.

- ✓ **Over 12 reps** – This can be a great range for beginners as it allows you to gain muscular endurance. Generally you are using lighter weight which allows you to hone in on form and make sure that you are completing exercises effectively and efficiently.

Even though you may want to stick within a certain rep range for your specific goals don't be afraid to complete a few sets in a different rep range. For example if you are working on gaining muscle your range is 8-12; don't be afraid to complete a few sets at a lower rep range (with a heavier weight) to develop more strength or a few sets with more reps (with a lighter weight) to work on endurance.

240) THE PERFECT REP!

'The perfect rep' or TEMPO should be the basis of your strength training where each repetition is completed with perfect form. I like the method referred to as compensatory acceleration training (CAT) which involves a fast positive (concentric) phase of contraction paired with a slower negative (eccentric) phase of contraction. The positive should be done explosively over a 1-2 second count, and the negative portion of the repetition should be done a little more slowly, over a 2-3 second count. When doing the explosive positive, you should decelerate before the end of the contraction so that you reduce stress on the joints and prepare your body for the slower negative phase of contraction. At the end of the negative phase, allow the rep to finish before you explode back into the positive. In other words, do not ever use momentum to move the weight. For example when doing a bench press lift the bar off of the rack and slowly lower it for a count of 2-3 down to your chest, take a subtle pause at the bottom and explode up to the top making your chest, triceps, and shoulders fire, then repeat the motion. The negative part of the motion is just as important (if not more) as the positive!

SETS: You have decided how many reps you want to do in a particular workout, but how many sets should you complete for each muscle group? If you are a beginner (been working out for less than 3 months 2-3 days a week), I would suggest 1-2 exercises per body part with 2-3 sets per muscle group to yield positive results. Remember more is NOT necessarily better! Do not push yourself too hard as you won't have ample time to repair your body. This will heighten your risk for injury and become OVERTRAINED: a condition where your muscles won't respond anymore to working out as they are in a constant catabolic (muscle breakdown) state. Follow this short guide below for general recommendations on how many sets you should do:

- ✓ 1-5 reps = 4-6 sets per body part.

- ✓ 6-8 reps = 3-5 sets per body part.

- ✓ 8-12 reps = 3-4 sets per body part.

- ✓ Over 12 reps = 2-3 sets per body part.

REST: The amount of rest between sets also depends on your workout and your ultimate goal. If your aim is to build muscular strength, this means that you will be doing a low amount of reps and high amount of sets. If this is your goal you will want to give yourself 3-4 minutes between sets to allow for proper recovery. If your goal is muscular endurance, you will be doing more reps at a lighter weight and fewer sets so the recovery period can be shorter, 30-60 seconds should do the trick!

You also have to think about what muscle it is that you are working out! For example, a set of weighted squats will be significantly harder than a bicep curl so vary your rest time according to the muscle as well. The last thing you want to do is not provide your body with sufficient rest as this will overwork the muscles and potentially cause an injury!

Full-Body Workouts

241) FILL YOUR WEEK WITH FULL BODY WORKOUTS!

'I don't have the time to work out!' is a complaint that I hear far too often. Full body workouts WORK because they are EFFICIENT! The benefits of a full body workout include:

1) Time efficiency – can be great to fit into a tight schedule; should be performed 2-3 times a week for no more than an hour each session.

2) Greater muscle recovery due to less stress.

3) Can prepare you for a sporting event/activity.

4) Will provide you with a metabolism spike.

5) Will increase muscle tissue.

6) Can be done at home.

7) Great for weight loss as you will be working ALL muscle groups at least twice a week.

Try one of these full body workouts, 2-3 days a week. If you are looking to get toned, 3-4 sets of 10-15 repetitions of EACH exercise will allow for muscular growth and endurance as you are both in the hypertrophy range (8-12) and in the endurance range (more than 12). If you want to add some muscle to your frame, perform 3-5 sets of 8-12 reps. Take NO LONGER than 30 seconds in between sets.

Example Schedule - Full Body Workout Program

SUNDAY	MONDAY	TUESDAY	WEDNESDAY	THURSDAY	FRIDAY	SATURDAY
Off	Workout 1	Cardio	Workout 2	Off	Workout 1	Cardio

This is an example schedule for a full body workout program which can be used for lean muscle gains, toning, and fat burning. The reps can be between 8-12 for more muscle building, 10-15 for toning, and 13-20 reps for toning and muscular endurance. Full body workouts should be done 2-3 days a week with a day's rest or cardio in between. You may do workout #1 for the week, Workout #2 for the week, or a combination of the both. Keep track of how much weight you use and go heavier if you can on each consecutive set going to failure (until you can't do any more reps). If something is too easy you can add more weight or if you don't have weights, slow the tempo down to create more tension on the muscles. Complete the first 3 exercises in a row (circuit A) with as little rest as possible. Take a 1-2 minute breather and repeat a total of three times. Then move on to circuit B for 3 times through, then circuit C.

Full Body Workout #1

For demonstrations of ALL exercises listed in this workout please visit my YouTube page: www.youtube.com/c/joeythurmanfit.

FULL BODY WORKOUT # 1 - EXERCISES	SET #1 (reps/weight)	SET #2 (reps/weight)	SET #3 (reps/weight)
Circuit A			
Crunches w/Tilt - 20-30 Reps			
Squats or Step Ups			
Flat-Bench Presses or Pushups			
Circuit B			

Back or Front Lunges			
Chin-ups or Rows			
Shoulder Press or Lateral Raises			
Circuit C			
Triceps Pushdowns or Kickbacks			
Curls with weights or Bands			
Standing Calf Raises			

Full Body Workout #2

For demonstrations of ALL exercises listed in this workout please visit my YouTube page: www.youtube.com/c/joeythurmanfit.

FULL BODY WORKOUT #2 - EXERCISES	SET #1 (reps/weight)	SET #2 (reps/weight)	SET #3 (reps/weight)
Circuit A			
Front or side Plank 30-60 seconds			
Leg Presses or Split Squats			
Side Lunge or Plie Squat			
Circuit B			
Incline Bench Press or Pushup			
Lat Pulldowns or Rows			
Shoulder Press or Lateral Raise			
Circuit C			
Triceps Extensions or Kickback			
Curls with weights or bands			
Standing Calf Raises			

Split-Body Routines

242) SPLIT IT UP FOR SUCCESS!

A split body workout can be done on 2 consecutive days, take a day off in between with rest or cardio, and finish your other 2 workouts for the week.

Example Schedule - 4 Day Split Body Routine

SUNDAY	MONDAY	TUESDAY	WEDNESDAY	THURSDAY	FRIDAY	SATURDAY
OFF	Workout #1	Workout #2	CARDIO	Workout #3	Workout #4	CARDIO

This is an example schedule for a 4 day split body workout program which can be used for lean muscle gains, toning, and fat burning. The reps can be between 8-12 for more muscle building, 10-15 for toning, and 13-20 reps for toning and muscular endurance. Split routine workouts should be done 3-5 days a week with your days off being cardio or rest days. Keep track of how much weight you use and go heavier if you can on each consecutive set going to failure (until you can't do any more reps). If something is too easy you can add more weight; if you don't have weights slow the tempo down to create more tension on the muscles. Complete the first 3 exercises in a row (circuit A) with as little rest as possible, take a 1-2 minute breather and repeat for a total of 3-5 times (only do 5 sets if you are an advanced lifter). Then move on to circuit B 3-5 times through, then circuit C. You may mix up the workout order but DON'T repeat the same muscle groups 2 days in a row! Muscles need time to rest and recover!

Workout #1 Chest, Shoulders, and Abs

For demonstrations of ALL exercises listed in this workout please visit my YouTube page: www.youtube.com/c/joeythurmanfit.

SPLIT BODY WORKOUT #1 - EXERCISES	SET #1 (reps/weight)	SET #2 (reps/weight)	SET #3 (reps/weight)
Circuit A			
Flat Bench Presses			
Incline Dumbbell Flys			
Dumbbell Presses			
Circuit B			
Lateral Raises			
Upright Rows			
Pushups			
Circuit C			
One-Arm Pushdowns			
Crunches - 20-30 Reps			
Plank – 30-60 Seconds			

Workout #2 Legs, Back, and Biceps

For demonstrations of ALL exercises listed in this workout please visit my YouTube page: www.youtube.com/c/joeythurmanfit.

SPLIT BODY WORKOUT #2 - EXERCISES	SET #1 (reps/weight)	SET #2 (reps/weight)	SET #3 (reps/weight)
Circuit A			
Squats			
Split Squats			
Ball Hamstring Curls			
Circuit B			
Standing Calf Raises			
Back or Front Lunge			
Rows			
Circuit C			
Seated Cable Rows or Pullups			
Barbell/Dumbbell Curls			
Alternating Dumbbell Curls			

Workout #3 Chest, Back, Biceps, Abs

For demonstrations of ALL exercises listed in this workout please visit my YouTube page: www.youtube.com/c/joeythurmanfit.

SPLIT BODY WORKOUT #3 - EXERCISES	SET #1 (reps/weight)	SET #2 (reps/weight)	SET #3 (reps/weight)
Circuit A			
Barbell Bench Press			
Standing Barbell/Dumbbell Curls			
Incline Dumbbell Presses			
Circuit B			
Lat Pulldown or Cable Rows			
One-Arm Dumbbell Rows			
Concentration Curls			
Circuit C			
Pullovers			
Hammer Curls			
Crunches - 20-30 Reps			
Leg Raises - 15-20 Reps			

Workout #4 Legs, Shoulders, and Triceps

For demonstrations of ALL exercises listed in this workout please visit my YouTube page: www.youtube.com/c/joeythurmanfit.

SPLIT BODY WORKOUT #4 - EXERCISES	SET #1 (reps/weight)	SET #2 (reps/weight)	SET #3 (reps/weight)
Circuit A			
Squats			
Split Squats			
Front Lunges			
Circuit B			
Plie Squats			
Standing Calf Raises			
Shoulder Press			
Lateral Raises			
Circuit C			
Upright Rows			
Dumbbell Shrugs			
Lying Triceps Extensions			

Interval Training

243) HIIT IT UP!

There's no doubt cardiovascular exercise benefits your health by improving heart health, mental health, joint support (if done properly), lowering risk of diabetes, and much more. However, the problem with consistent steady state cardio, especially if you don't resistance train, is you will not develop a well-defined physique. I use the following example to get my point across; if you look like a large pear and do nothing but steady state cardio, you may lose weight, but you will simply just look like a smaller pear without a lot of muscle definition. Believe me, I like going for a long steady run in the summer to get a good sweat; and mostly to take my shirt off to get a tan; but I still do interval training and weight training to provide the stimulus to really sculpt my body into what my Theia (aunt in Greek) Martha calls me...Hercules!

So let's take cardio up a notch and talk about another method that may be even more superior to steady state cardio. I'm talking about interval training, or High Intensity

Interval Training (HIIT), which in my opinion, and many other health professionals, is the BEST form of cardio. It gives you the highest amount of benefits in the shortest amount of time; and isn't this the reason you are reading this book in the first place? Just compare an Olympic sprinter verse an Olympic marathon runner; their frames are much different where the distance runner is incredibly thin and the sprinter has well-developed muscles that can be seen from the top of the grandstands!

Intervals are a form of cardio where you perform an intense exercise as hard as you can; such as running sprints, swimming fast, jumping rope, weight training, or riding hard on a bike. The idea behind HIIT is to elevate your heart rate for a brief period (even walking for beginners), followed by resting for a given period (at least the amount of the time you were sprinting). For example: you can interval train in a 1:1 work to rest ratio (sprint for 30sec, rest for 30sec), a 1:2 ratio (sprint for 30sec, rest for 1min), a 1:3 ratio (sprint for 30 sec, rest for 1.5min), and so forth.

Intervals are for more than extreme athletes and weekend warriors; they truly are for EVERYONE and should be performed by everyone in some capacity, but you must adapt it to your individual needs…be smart here people! Here is what interval training can do for you:

✓ Intervals have been shown to **REPAIR your metabolism**, by reducing inflammation and forcing the body to improve its ability to use and burn energy [21].

✓ **They will give you Abs** - Everyone wants a six pack that just won't quit, but they waste their time doing sit-ups all day long. Here it is for you plain and simple, if you want to see your abs, or want better abs, you need to lose the layer of fat that is covering them up. Weight training and interval training are the best way to lose your love handles and melt belly fat fast.

✓ **Give you Lean Legs** - Intervals are amazing for burning fat all over your body and not just your stomach. Intervals will tone your legs including your butt, quads, hamstrings, and calves as long as the intervals you are doing are lower body intensive like running or biking. In one study, young men who did 20 minutes of bike intervals for 3 months increased leg musculature by 0.5 kg, while losing 2 kg of body fat (that's almost 4.5 pounds of fat!). Sprints enhance protein synthesis pathways by as much as 230 percent and increase the size and strength of fast twitch muscle fibers [22].

✓ **Improved Body Composition** – Weight training and interval training are the two ways to increase the body's ability to burn calories throughout the day. This is called Excess Post-Exercise Oxygen Consumption (EPOC). If you strictly perform endurance style cardio you can lose muscle in the long run because your body starts to become catabolic; a state where you burn through muscle tissue and lower your metabolism. Adding muscle tissue through weights and intervals will elevate your metabolism for days…and for a lifetime [24]!

✓ **Improves fat burning!** – Normally the first macronutrient your body uses as energy is carbohydrates. 'Metabolic flexibility' is known as your body being able to burn fat as energy before carbohydrates, but most people don't have this capability. In order to achieve metabolic flexibility, you need to drop down your carbohydrate levels in order for your body to use fat as energy, but this has been shown to only work for people who are already lean and healthy. For overweight people, intervals have been shown to increase their metabolic flexibility. For example in one recent study, doing four 30-second sprints on a cycle ergometer increased fat burning by 75 percent, 75%! In fact, the elevated use of fat for fuel was sustained for at least two hours after the workout.

✓ **Prevent Diabetes and fix your metabolism.** –Numerous studies show intervals improve insulin health in the young, old, overweight, diabetic, and folks with metabolic syndrome. When you build muscle, you increase the receptiveness of the muscles to insulin and their demand for glucose. In other words, your muscles can utilize sugars for energy as opposed to elevating blood sugar levels and being stored as fat.

✓ **Lower Blood Pressure & Improve Heart Health** – Traditional cardio should be considered second rate as studies show interval training demonstrates better cardiovascular outcomes by improving heart health and lowering blood pressure. A 2011 study in overweight women showed increased stroke volume and a reduced heart rate both at rest and during training after 4 weeks of cycle sprints.

- ✓ **Better coordination** - Intervals improve coordination by working the fast twitch muscle fibers of the body that are responsible for reaction time and prime the nervous system to react quicker. Maybe it's time to get Grandma to do some interval training (at the least the walking kind).

- ✓ **Higher Testosterone & Growth Hormone** - Intervals increase testosterone levels in men allowing them to get more muscular and increase growth hormone (gh) in women which helps with fat burning and tissue repair.

- ✓ **Makes you smarter!** - We all hear that exercise is good for your body and mind but intervals have been shown to actually improve your brain capacity by raising adrenaline hormones that stimulate the brain and boost neurotransmitter function in the brain such as dopamine.

- ✓ **Get More Powerful and increase endurance!** - When you are powerful you can express your strength quickly and explosively. The muscles stretch and shorten at an explosive rate and create power known as the stretch-shortening-cycle. This can be done with any all-out exercise on a track by doing sprints, running stairs, riding a stationary bike and even some forms of weight training at an all-out effort. When you become more powerful through intervals you will make your regular endurance exercises seem much easier. All of a sudden your Sunday run will become a jog in the park...ha!

- ✓ Doing sprints **increases the amount of glycogen** (stored carbs) that can be utilized by your muscles, increases the body's ability to remove waste products, and increases mental toughness! If you can get through an interval training session your body will love you for it and everything else in life will seem easy!

Ok, Ok, enough of me telling you why you need to do intervals, here are some hacks on how to interval train with the best of 'em!

244) INTERVALS FOR TRUE BEGINNERS!

If you are out of shape, or simply new to working out, HIIT training doesn't have to be performed like Usain Bolt in the Olympics! Start with simple run and walk intervals (or cycling, swimming, etc.).

- ✓ *How:* warm up with a walk outside or on a treadmill for about 5 minutes. Once your muscles are warmed up, run for about 30 seconds even if this isn't technically a "sprint" for you, it will seem like one. Once the 30 seconds is up if you are on a treadmill bring it down to a walk or if you are outside simply slow down and start walking. Walk for one minute to 2 minutes and go back into your run. Repeat this for a total of 25 minutes, cool down with a walk, stretch, and/or foam roll; then enjoy a nutritious post workout meal. Do these 2-3 days a week and each time try to run faster and/or cut down you rest time until you can get to a 1:2 or 1:1 ratio.

245) INTERVALS FOR METABOLIC CONDITIONS!

If you are obese, have diabetes, elderly, have high blood pressure, or have arthritis give this a shot. This will get you to adapt to exercise, gain energy, and lose fat.

- ✓ *How:* Start with a brisk walk for 3 minutes as fast as you can (get those arms moving) and then walk slowly for 3 minutes. Continue this for 25-30 minutes and increase your intensity each time!

246) 8's AND 12's!

For beginners to experts. This will help your lose fat, improve insulin health, increase power, and build lean muscle tissue.

- ✓ *How:* Make sure you are warmed up and perform 8 seconds of work and then take 12 seconds of active rest by walking or slowing down (if you are biking, swimming, etc.). Do this for a total of 20 minutes for a total of 60 times through.

247) 1:1 LONG DURATION INTERVALS!

If you really want to increase your aerobic capacity and fat burning potential this is for you! I warn you this is NOT for the beginner or the weak!

✓ *How:* Get on a track, in a pool, on a bike, etc. Perform your sprint about 85-90% of your maximal effort for a total of two minutes. Take a 2 minute breather, and repeat for a total of 4-6 times. This is a very intense workout and can be done 2-4 times a week. Work your way up to 6 rounds and remember to push yourself, get plenty of rest, and proper nutrition.

248) SUPER 8's!

If you want a quick HIIT workout and really want to reap the fat loss and other benefits try Super 8's! No, this is not something superman does, although you may feel like superman (or superwoman) afterwards.

✓ *How:* Warmup for a few minutes and then perform a sprint as fast as you can for 30 seconds; this should be so fast where you can't do another second! Take a 1 minute to 1.5 minute breather (only take 1 minute if you are advanced) so you have a 1:2 or 1:3 work to rest ratio)) and then repeat 7 more times for a total of 8 rounds! You will be done with your workout in 12-14 minutes (not including your warmup and cool down). Do this 2-3 days and week and after a few weeks you will be thanking me for how amazing you look, and more importantly feel!

249) DO A COMPLETE 180!

This is a workout I came up with a couple of years ago and is a mix between maximal heart rate aerobic conditioning and anaerobic (muscular) stimulation! The workout is called the Complete 180 because you complete180 reps as safely and as fast as you possibly can! This workout is meant to be done anywhere, anytime, and by anyone!

✓ *How:* There are 3 different exercises that will challenge every muscle in your body as well as your cardiovascular system. This workout should be done with a fast tempo but under control. If you need a break at any point take it, compose yourself and continue with the rest of the exercises

The first exercise is a push-up with an oblique knee tuck (or peeing on the fire hydrant). Start with your hands about shoulder width apart, slowly lower yourself while keeping your abs engaged until your chest reaches the ground and drive up through your palms to squeeze your chest, shoulders, and triceps. Once your arms are locked out at the top position bring one leg slightly off of the ground and tuck your knee toward the same shoulder to engage your obliques, repeat the movement with the other leg and go back to the push-up. The first round will be 16 reps of this movement.

After the push-up flip your body around so that your chest is facing the sky and you are on your palms and the soles of your feet (called a bridge tuck). Keep your hips up to engage your butt and pull one knee towards your chest to contract your abs. Alternate sides until you reach 16 reps each leg for the first round.

The last exercise in the first round is a split jump. Start with your feet staggered (in a lunging position) and jump upward so that you can alternate the leg that lands to the front of your body. Make sure to have a soft landing so that your knee and hip form about a 90 degree angle. Repeat so that you compete 16 reps each leg.

This is the first circuit in the 180 workout, take a few deep breaths and repeat the push-ups, bridge tucks, and split jumps for 14 reps each, then 12 reps, 10 reps, and finally 8 reps each so that you will complete 180 reps in no time!

This workout will leave you feeling accomplished, ready for the day, and very exhausted! *Note: you can do any exercises you choose as long as they are 3 different muscle groups; get creative and get in shape in no time!

*For demonstrations of the Complete 180 Workout please visit my YouTube page: www.youtube.com/c/joeythurmanfit.

*For complete exercise routines delivered straight to your email and smart device check out the Renovation Plans on my website www.TheLifestyleRenovation.com

'Exercise for Life' Hacks

Now it's time to have a look at some other tips and exercises that will help you on your way to glory!

250) ALWAYS COOL DOWN!
Cooling down is equally important as it can help to resume the body back to a normal temperature. A simple cool down can help to remove lactic acid that builds up in the

muscles; which means that you won't ache as much later on! A five minute walk on the treadmill followed by foam rolling/stretching will do the trick.

251) THROW AWAY THE AB BELT AND SIT-UP MACHINE!

What, that thing that shocks my stomach will not transform my beer belly into rock hard abs? Oh, if only it were that easy, but truth be told, you cannot SPOT reduce the fat away, whether it's with an ab belt or a sit-up machine. If you want to lose your belly, doing crunches all day long will not get rid of your stomach fat and magically turn you into Brad Pitt in Fight Club. Sure doing crunches can help, but it needs to be in conjunction with an effective workout routine and a nutrition plan so you can lose body fat that is covering your abs! Eat clean and follow the tips in this book and you will start to see your abs and you can throw away your "couch fitness" devices! "Couch fitness" enthusiasts, like to think they can get in shape simply by sitting on the couch and doing a few crunches using a magical product! Truth is, you can't, and all you're doing is spending money on products that don't work.

252) ACTIVITY TRACKER!

There are so many activity trackers available now that can track everything from our workouts to our sleep. Lots of these trackers input the data in an app that can log your food, water intake, calorie burn, heart rate (now on your wrist which is much less annoying than the chest strap) and more! I just love the technology now; you can literally track everything you are doing and encourage yourself to MOVE more! Common brands are the Fitbit, Jawbone, Garmin, iWatch, and hundreds of others! Pick the one that is most convenient to your lifestyle. If you are a runner make sure one can track your distance, pace, time and log it seamlessly. If you like to swim, make sure the watch is WATER Proof not just water resistant. Do your research and just because something is more expensive doesn't mean it's better for you!

253) HOLD THE CONTRACTION!

When working out it isn't simply enough to "do" the exercise. If you are completing a bicep curl you want to feel your biceps working otherwise what is the point? If you don't feel the muscle you are trying to develop actively working do you think you are going to get your desired results? No! Focus on squeezing the muscle through the entire contraction. On a bicep curl, focus on making a muscle on the way up (the positive) part of the motion squeezing at the top, and control down (the negative) part of the motion making sure you feel your biceps control the weight down. This can be done for any movement from biceps, to legs, to abs. Focus on the muscle you are working and squeeze it like you are walking down a beach naked, every muscle will be tight to impress whoever you have your eyes on!

254) THE FIRST MONTH IS THE HARDEST!

If you stick to your schedule for the first month, the rest should follow pretty easily. Make exercise your hobby! It is very easy to give up in the first few weeks but DON'T, stick to it and soon it will just become second nature!

255) RESISTANCE TRAINING, RESISTING AGING!

Is exercise important for maintaining our youth? OF COURSE it is! That is a well-known statement full of truth, but did you know that hours and hours of cardio can actually have the opposite effect. You need to make sure that you mix it up a bit; introduce some resistance training to help burn fat and build muscle! It will also help to tighten skin and decrease the appearance of cellulite [1]! STOP RESISTING RESISTANCE TRAINING!

256) ONE MINUTE A DAY!

If you are a complete beginner, start with a small run (as your workout or after your resistance training)! On the first day, run for a minute, walk for 29min; on day two, run for 2 minutes and walk for 28min, until eventually on day thirty, you will be running for the full half hour! This is a great method to slowly increase your running capacity.

257) REST DAYS ARE VITAL!

A lot of people burn themselves out within two weeks of a program because they don't allow themselves a day off. Days off can be just as important as workout days because your body needs to repair all the muscles and tendons that you have strained while exercising!

258) TALK WHILE RUNNING (IF YOU'RE WITH SOMEONE)!

Talking while running can help to regulate your breathing making your running more efficient! When we run in silence, we tend to place A LOT of concentration on our breathing when it should be natural. I'm not suggesting talking to yourself if you don't have a running buddy (although it would help).

259) WORKOUT BEFORE A BAD MEAL!

We ALL do this, and yes even a "celebrity" fitness expert such as myself! We know we have a bad meal full of delicious sweets and fattening food about to come our way with friends or family that will be all but impossible to stay away from. Yes, you can do everything in your power not to eat this bad meal, but you know that no matter what, that food is going into your belly! So what do you do, burn it off later? No! Try to burn it off before! What? If you work out hard before a bad meal with weight training or some interval training like sprints, jumping rope, or playing a sport, your body will likely utilize the bad food that you eat to replenish your muscle cells, repair your body, and less likely be stored as fat...score!

260) PLAYLIST AS LONG AS YOUR WORKOUT!

Music is shown to increase the efficiency and workload of your exercise routine and can be a great way to take the focus off of the workout itself. Make a playlist of your favorite tunes and blast them out if you are at home (earphones if in the gym, of course, otherwise people may get annoyed) to help you during your workout. Make the playlist as long as you want to work out. That way you don't have to keep checking the time; you will finish when the music finishes! *Side note, music is great to listen to in the gym, but don't be the one who is singing along to the song; people pay for a gym membership to work out and not to listen to your karaoke version of Celine, thanks!

261) DRINKING GAME!

I'm sorry if I got your hopes up, but this one won't be involving any alcohol (obviously). Every time one of your favorite TV character says his famous catchphrase, you can drop and do ten push-ups, squats, or sit-ups followed by a drink of water. Get creative, have fun, and getting healthy and fit will come with it.

262) KEEP A GYM BAG IN THE CAR!

You never know when inspiration may strike or when you have an hour or two to kill before you have to go back to work. Keep a bag in the car with workout clothes, a towel, deodorant and anything else you need so you are always ready!

263) GET A PET!

Our furry friends are like children, they constantly need love, attention, and to be taken for walks. Dogs in particular love and need exercise so why not take the opportunity to walk the dog or maybe even jog with the dog instead of letting someone else do it! Soon man's best friend will become man's life saver!

264) EXERCISE WHILE WORKING!

It can be EXTREMELY harmful to be sitting in one place all day yet many of us with office jobs do it on a daily basis. However, there are ways to exercise at your desk; without even having to stand up. For example, sit up in your chair, tense your abs and raise your legs up so they are even with your hips! Do this around 15 times for each leg! Get creative when you are walking down the hall; do some walking lunges, take the stairs to the meeting, or even challenge your friend to a race to the lunch room; now that would be fun!

265) POSITIVE THINKING AND TALKING!

Research has shown that thinking positively as well as talking positively can help with how well you perform during exercise. Next time you are going for a new personal best bench press, make sure you are with someone who believes in you [3]! If you work out alone, harness the power of visualization and verbalization. Visualize yourself lifting that weight and then talk it out!

266) WATERPROOF YOURSELF!

'Oh, I was about to go running but then it started raining!' – NOT AN EXCUSE! Buy yourself some waterproof clothes so you can run in all weathers. You can even get a waterproof cover for your phone/mp3 player!

267) PAY FOR CLASSES UP FRONT!

Paying for exercise classes or a personal trainer up front will immediately increase the likelihood of you attending because you will be wasting money if you don't! Money makes the world go round! It's wise to not lose money you have worked hard for; so it's best to go to that spin class!

268) USE TECHNOLOGY!

We live in an age now where EVERYTHING can be found on the internet, from a bird on a skateboard to 'how to make a bookcase'. Use this to your advantage! Look up great websites and even videos on YouTube to find some workouts. Maybe you can't afford a gym membership, the gym is too far away, or you lack time. YouTube is FULL of home workout tutorials! Better yet, check out my YouTube channel https://www.youtube.com/c/joeythurmanfit for great exercise tips and workout ideas.

269) PLAN EVERYTHING AHEAD!

I mean EVERYTHING! The more we plan the night before, the more likely we are to go ahead with our plans. Plan and prep your meals so you don't have an excuse to eat fast food. Pack a workout bag with your clothes, equipment, etc. Even plan your work outfit the day before to create a bit more time in the am for some push-ups and squats. Remove all the possible excuses that could be used!

270) FEELING ILL? TRY ANYWAY!

If you are feeling under the weather, give your planned session a 10-minute trial to see how you feel. Exercise naturally puts us in a better mood and it is likely after 10 minutes, you will want to carry on!

271) MAKE USE OF VIDEO GAMES!

If you're going to play a video game, why not exercise at the same time. If you have an exercise bike, hop on while playing your game, you will find that you start to pedal faster during intense or important moments! You can also make the video game your exercise. Get an interactive game where you can use a wireless remote like the Wii or PlayStation move to marry your love for video games with burning calories!

272) LONG PHONE CONVERSATION? WALK!

If you see a phone call coming through and you know that it will be a long one (maybe your mom is calling to check up on you or your friend is calling for some gossip from the weekend), why not go for a walk? This will be MUCH better for you than sitting down! If all you are doing is talking, why not exercise at the same time?

273) EVERY LITTLE BIT HELPS!

If you started your work out and for some reason need to stop during your cardio or your weight training session, ITS OK! Sometimes life happens and pulls you away from what you want to do and you have to take care of pressing issues right there and then. Do not worry if you only got a mile or a few sets in. You can finish the workout later in the day or make up for it the next day! Now if you stopped your workout because of a lame excuse, like having to water your plants, then yes, you should absolutely feel guilty!!

274) EXERCISE IN THE SHOWER!

Maybe today is the day where you have a full day from start to finish and you really don't have enough time to work out, make the most of your time in the shower! See how many squats or wall push-ups you can do getting clean! (I got this one from my wife. I laughed the first time, and each time after that, but it truly can be an efficient use of your time!) But before you partake, be sure your shower has a nonslip grip floor to reduce risk of injury.

275) SQUAT OR PUSH-UPS BEFORE MEALS!

Just 90 seconds of either exercise can be enough to trigger your body to send the nutrients from the meal to your muscles instead of being stored as fat! EASY! Just set your watch and bang out 90 seconds of squats, pushups, or a combination of both (or opt for lunges and pullups).

276) WARM UP YOUR BUTT!

When running, it is normal to experience some back ache, this means that your butt is not taking the shock of your steps. Back lunges or split squats before a run should be enough to get the glute muscles firing to absorb the shock as you run, taking the pressure off of your back.

277) EXERCISE DURING COMMERCIAL BREAKS!

So your favorite TV program is on and you wouldn't miss it for the world! Any other program you would skip for a workout but not this one! You can still make the most of the situation by writing down some small exercises on scraps of paper or note cards. As soon as a commercial starts, pull a piece of paper from the stack and complete the exercise that is written down! This can be anything that will get the blood pumping around your body; sit-ups, push-ups, ab crunches, 100 jumping jacks, 20 jump squats, 20 burpees, and maybe even holding a plank for the ENTIRE break (challenge yourself)!

278) USE THE STAIRS!

The elevator is too easy, right? All you have to do is walk in, push a button and wait. BORING! Take the stairs and get some extra exercise into your day! Even if it is just one floor, it still gets the blood pumping (you shouldn't be taking an elevator for one floor anyway). Just walking upstairs for two minutes can burn 25 calories, while using an elevator burns... you guessed it, ZERO!

279) PARK FAR AWAY!

This follows the same logic as using the stairs. Parking further away from your destination will allow you to get more exercise. Also, write down EVERYHWHERE you drive and reconsider whether it's necessary. Driving has become a habit and we tend to just take the car because it is convenient, but do we really need it for 3 minute journey to the store? PROBABLY NOT!

280) 'I WILL JUST WORKOUT OVER THE WEEKEND'!

Nope, not going to work! You cannot undo five days of not working out with just two days of exercise. You will be better off switching that around and working out during the week and taking the weekend off! How about becoming a WEEKDAY WARRIOR!?

281) TREE CLIMBING!

Everyone loved being a kid, right? Playing in the park, riding your bike, climbing trees! Why does this have to change? Next time you are in the park, inject a bit of energy by climbing a tree, playing on the swings, or maybe you can have a race with a friend (or your child); just don't knock any kids over in the process.

282) WASH YOUR OWN CAR!

It is very easy nowadays to get our car cleaned for us at a car wash, but why not save money and burn calories doing it ourselves? We can burn 6 calories A MINUTE just by cleaning our own car; so a half an hour manual car wash has just burned 180 CALORIES! Cleaning your own car can also be therapeutic; you can put your iPod on and listen to some of your favorite music and relax!

283) TRACK YOUR STEPS!

With advancements of technology over the years, pedometers are now both affordable and small. The first time you wear a pedometer you will be surprised by how many steps you take in a day, but set a goal that is even higher than that.

284) OUT GOES THE OFFICE CHAIR!

Try swapping your office chair with an exercise ball! We tend to slouch or lean to one side when sitting on a chair which can lead to a number of injuries! Sitting on an exercise ball requires good posture which activates the core muscles of the abdomen, back AND hips!

Just remember to keep good posture while sitting on the ball as slouching negates the benefits.

285) WEIGHTS FIRST, CARDIO SECOND!

Most beginners tend to start their workouts with cardio; STOP! It is a much better idea to do your weight training FIRST. This way your muscles haven't already tired out when you try that first squat! Another added bonus is doing your cardio after weight training will burn more body fat! The reason for this is weight training burns up glycogen (the storage form of carbohydrates). So when you do cardio afterwards, you will pull from your fat stores to provide energy for you cardio session.

286) BE VAIN!

Gym-goers and weight lifters get a lot of flak for watching themselves in the mirror when exercising, but laugh no more! It's not necessarily because they like watching themselves or because they are posing (although I do, ha!); it is because they are watching their FORM! If you are looking in a mirror while you lift, you can mind your posture which maximizes results and prevents injury!

287) FARMERS WALK!

This is so simple yet SO effective. Try starting or ending your workout by simply walking around with a heavy object, you can use one or two of your dumbbells, a kettlebell or anything else you may find in your house! Have the weights either by your side (like you are carrying suitcases) or holding the weight high up on your chest. Remember to keep your chest up, abs engaged, and breathe naturally. Do this for a couple of minutes to work on your grip, posture, and core stability.

288) KETTLEBELL SWINGS!

This exercise will work out your WHOLE BODY and will get your heart pumping like never before! Pick a weight that you are comfortable with. Squat down to pick up the weight and drive upwards with your arms to swing the weight in front of your chest with your arms extended. Keep your abs engaged and squeeze your butt to keep your back from taking over; let the weight guide your arms down until the kettlebell is below your butt and swing back upwards. Feel the burn all over your body but especially in the legs, back, abs and shoulders! Start with a couple of sets of 10. Over time, gradually increase until you are able to complete 100 swings in less than 10 minutes with minimal rest between sets (about 30 seconds to a minute). When you feel like you have mastered that weight, INCREASE IT!

289) LESS REST!

Challenge yourself by reducing the amount of rest you give yourself between sets of an exercise. This will make the workout more intense and extremely challenging. If you normally have 30 seconds rest, reduce it to 25 or even 20; with the eventual aim of reaching 15 seconds between sets!

290) ACTIVE REST!

You have a busy schedule and don't have a lot of time for exercise; that means you should choose either cardio OR weights! NOPE! Let me introduce to you something called active rest where you complete cardio exercise IN BETWEEN sets of weights. You could jump rope, do high knees, or maybe even hold a plank in between sets! This will definitely get intense and challenging, but will be totally worth it. Nothing better than feeling like a machine after you kicked active rest's butt!

291) DON'T GET TOO COMFORTABLE!

If you are starting to finish your sets easily, that's great. It's an indication you are getting stronger, but that DOESN'T mean you should stop there. Keep varying your workout to keep challenging yourself. If you are completing your ten reps easily, it's important to increase the weight you are using; even if it means dropping to 6-8 reps until you can do the full set!

292) STRAP THEM UP!

Investing in some good straps could really benefit your workout! When working on our back we tend to lose grip and maybe finish the set before we really need to. Straps will help to secure our grip and help us to push out a couple more reps which will increase our muscle growth!

293) QUALITY NOT QUANTITY!

The quality of our workout is FAR more important than the quantity. We often feel like we are not doing enough in the gym when our friends tell us that they spent over two hours in there. Two hours is definitely overkill...especially if most of their time is spent resting and socializing...you know who you are! This is not going to be you! You can do an efficient workout in an hour. Use the tips learned so far to create an intense workout so you can work hard in no time flat and get on with the rest of your day!

294) KEEP A NATURAL BACK!

Form is vital, so keep your back at a neutral position (with shoulder back and chest up) when lifting weights. If you are forcing a position that isn't comfortable for your body, you could end up slipping a disc or experiencing another permanent injury; and that is the LAST thing we need when changing our life and getting fit!

295) BURNOUT SETS!

This is one of my favorite things to have clients do towards the end of their workouts and I know it's their LEAST favorite (but extremely beneficial). For example: if you are doing a leg workout finish your day with a set of back lunges for as many as you a can, or step ups on a bench for a minute. If you are doing chest finish with a set of pushups or plate presses until you reach a 100, get crazy, get creative, but be SAFE!

296) MAXIMUM HEART RATE!

Working out your maximum heart rate can be useful when completing high-intensity training! It can help you work out efficiently and safely. The old way of calculating maximum heart rate is 220 - your age. The most recent and thought to be the most accurate way to work this out is '211 – (your age x 0.64)'.

- ✓ **Fat Burning Zone:** 60-70% of your max HR is known as the 'fat burning zone'; where up to 85% of your calories burned are fat.

- ✓ **Aerobic Zone:** 70-80% of your max HR. This zone improves your functional capacity, the number and size of your blood vessels, increase lung capacity and respiratory rate, and benefits your heart; allowing you to exercise longer before becoming fatigued. You're metabolizing fats and carbohydrates at about a 50-50 rate which means both are burning at the same ratio. If you were to be in a fat burning zone for 10min and an aerobic zone for 10min, you will burn more overall calories in the aerobic zone.

- ✓ **Anaerobic Threshold Zone:** 80-90% of your maximum HR. This zone is reached by working extremely hard. You will get fitter and faster as your heart rate increases you cross from aerobic to anaerobic training (without sufficient oxygen). Your heart cannot pump enough blood and oxygen to supply the exercising muscles to a full extent so they respond by continuing to contract anaerobically.

✓ **Top End/Redline Zone:** 90-100% of your maximum HR. This is the equivalent to running as fast as you possibly can, most often used during interval training. You will not be able to maintain this pace longer than a minute or two; if you can you might be an Olympian! Be careful in this zone, that's why HIIT (intervals) are so great, you can reach your max heart rate briefly, drop it down, then get back up and go again!

297) FORCED REPS!

KEEP GOING! Forced reps are proven to help you MASSIVELY! People who push those last few forced reps out had growth hormone levels 4,000% higher than people who didn't! 4,000%!!! Of course, it goes without saying that we shouldn't go over the top with this and 'over train' or possibly injure ourselves but 2-3 extra reps could work wonders! Make sure to have a spotter or use a machine when doing forced reps for safety.

298) THINK ABOUT THE MUSCLE!

Thinking about the muscle that you are working can actually increase muscle activity in that area. Sounds crazy but it is completely true! For example, when doing bicep curls, concentrate on your biceps rather than where the beautiful brunette you were watching went!

299) MIX UP YOUR REP SPEED!

Switch up the speed of your reps to maximize your growth opportunities. Our fast and slow twitch fibers react differently to different exercises, and more importantly, different speeds of exercises. Faster reps tend to increase our muscle strength whereas slower reps increase our muscle mass! So, keep your muscles guessing and vary the rep speed often!

300) TREADMILL CHALLENGE!

Sometimes running on the treadmill can be boring so why not make it a little more challenging by taking some weights on there with you! It goes without saying that you shouldn't run at a fast pace on the treadmill with weights as it's a recipe for disaster. Set the speed to a brisk walk and start to perform basic exercises such as bicep curls or shoulder presses. This will challenge your body, but will be TOTALLY worth it!

301) STRENGTHEN YOUR RUNS!

You have just finished a decent run, whether it was on a treadmill or outside, but don't rest yet. You can strengthen your quads, glutes and hamstrings by completing a quick set of wall sits; this will improve your speed and endurance. A few sets of wall sits after a run can benefit you greatly. If you are unaware of what a wall sit entails here's how you do it: stand with your back against a wall, feet shoulder-width apart and slowly squat until your knees are at 90 degrees. Try to hold this for 20-30 seconds EACH TIME and feel the burn! *You can also try this before your run to activate the muscles in your legs and really feel every stride!

302) SNOW IS FALLING!

Time to pay the young lad next door to shovel the snow, NO! Why not do it yourself? Besides burning nearly 400 calories an hour, it will help to significantly boost muscle strength and endurance. Be careful not to overload the shovel each time and bend with your knees (not your back); otherwise you will cause some serious damage which isn't what we are after!

303) DOUBLE JUMP ROPE!

If you incorporate the 'double turn' you can burn around 25 CALORIES PER MINUTE! First, get into the rhythm of the normal jump, then when you start to feel comfortable, jump twice as high but keep your wrists turning at the same speed (if not, a little faster). The main aim of this is for the rope to pass underneath you twice before you land again. It may take some practice but once you get used to it this can be a REALLY efficient fat-burning exercise; as you can burn over 100 calories in less than five minutes.

304) JUMP THOSE BOXES!

You can really shape up your hamstrings, quads and glutes, improve leg strength, and improve stamina by completing box jumps. At the gym, you can start with a shorter box to get the hang of it and add more boxes (or use a taller one) each time. At home, a sturdy object that can hold your weight (like a bench) will also do the trick. Start by standing in front of the box and perform an explosive jump to pounce upwards on top of the box; step down and repeat this 15-20 times for maximum benefit!

305) DO YOUR CRUNCHES PROPERLY!

It can be easy to relax your abs on the way back down from a crunch but you can lose up to 50% performance by relaxing half-way through. So be sure to maintain the contraction on the way down to feel the full effect and get the maximum benefit!

306) KAYAK OR MIMIC KAYAKING!

Kayaking can be a GREAT exercise when working towards a flatter stomach because the majority of the energy used comes from your core! If you don't have access to a kayak center (let's face it, not all of us do!), you can replicate the same exercise using an exercise band. First, loop the band around a fixed object like a table leg or something of that caliber. Next, sit down on the floor with your legs extended with a slight bend at the knee. Grab one end of the band in each hand and rotate your torso from side to side. Try doing three sets of two minutes each and increase when you feel comfortable.

307) WHEN TO BREATHE?

This sounds like a silly question right? 'I just breathe naturally, I don't think about it;' well, start thinking about it more as it may help you out. Especially when running, we should exhale on ALTERNATE feet, this prevents adding extra stress to just one side of the body and can help to reduce the risk of cramps!

308) THE INCH WORM!

This is a nice and easy exercise that you can do on a DAILY BASIS especially as a warmup before resistance training! This will get the heart rate pumping and will target many muscle groups and give your hamstrings a good stretch. Start in a standing position, bend down and put both hands on the floor close to your toes and slowly 'walk' your hands forward until you are in the basic push-up position. Now complete one single push-up (this part is optional and more challenging). Finally, walk your hands back to your toes and stand up straight. Complete these in sets of 10!

309) HIP BRIDGES!

Who knew that lying down could be so effective? Lie down with your knees bent and feet flat on the floor. Slowly and gently raise your hips from the floor by lifting your hips and torso while your shoulders and heels stay flat on the ground. Be sure to squeeze your butt at the top.

FINISHING TOUCHES

Travel

What are we supposed to do when we travel and our daily routine gets shaken up with a new area flooded with new restaurants and new temptations? How can you still maintain healthy eating habits and stay fit? Surely, it's impossible? NO, definitely not! It is a common misconception that you can't eat healthy and stay fit when travelling the world. Yes, it is HARDER to be healthy when you are traveling, but that is NO excuse as long as you prepare ahead of time!

310) HOLIDAY ACTIVITIES!

So you have worked hard all year and now you have earned a week away in the sun, but that doesn't mean that the exercising has to stop. Normally, hotels and vacation resorts run all sorts of activities that you can get involved in so why not try that hiking or snorkeling excursion that is offered?

311) EAT WELL!

Well this sounds obvious right? Some people come to me and say that they couldn't find anywhere healthy to eat and I ask one simple question 'How hard did you look?' Did you spend time researching restaurants, grocery stores, or farmers markets in the area? The truth is that you will always be able to find healthy food wherever you go, it just depends how willing you are to research to find your best options. Go to the local market, pick up some foods that you haven't tried before, this way you are experiencing the culture but still eating healthy. You can even call down to room service and order something that may not be on the menu (grilled chicken salad or veggie omelet). More often than not a hotel or restaurant will be more than happy to accommodate…it doesn't hurt to ask!

312) SLEEP WELL!

We sometimes get caught up in this notion that we don't have to look after our bodies when travelling as we can fix it when we get home; that's a load of crap! By the time you get home from your trip the damage has already been done. Sleep is included in this, sitting around a campfire until the early hours of the morning, or partying the night away may sound tempting, but trust in that you WILL pay for it! You have to remember that your sleep is vital! You have learned how important sleep is in the 'sleep' section; it has an impact when you travel as well. Lack of sleep while you travel will end up altering your sleeping pattern. Upon returning home, your trip "hang-over" may last for days impeding on your everyday life (and workouts). Get a good 7/8 hours of sleep per night!

313) FIND MOTIVATION!

I completely accept that finding motivation to work out when travelling is a lot harder than when at home, but it is possible. If you have been working out consistently at home (I hope so) you don't want all of that hard work to go to waste! You have to find self-motivation as there is no one else that can do it for you. Tell yourself how good you are going to feel for staying healthy while away; focus on the positive aspects of staying the course.

314) RUN ON THE FIRST DAY!

Going out running on the first day when you arrive in a new place can be a GREAT way of getting to know the new surroundings. You can explore the local area; find restaurants that you may want to try, and find fun activities to do. Oh and if you aren't up for running you can speed walk (or ride a bike) your way around town… remember, no excuses!

315) GO TO THE PARK!

When travelling, you are more than likely staying in a hotel which doesn't really lend much room for exercise. You can always take a little trip down to the local park (or any open space) and move your workout there instead. You will benefit from the fresh air and it allows you to be creative with what the park has to offer. Monkey bars are a great tool for a workout! Become a kid again and 'monkey around!'

316) MOVE ABOUT THE CABIN!

You can spend hours on trains, planes, buses and other modes of transport that involves you sitting in one place for hours on end while you move from one place to the next. Standing up and warming your muscles becomes VITAL in this scenario! You need to keep the blood flowing to your tissues to remain lose. Too much time in one position can actually lead to Deep Vein Thrombosis as blood clots, and I know you don't want that! I recommend taking a walk up and down the aisle (when the seatbelt alert is off) or marching in place in your seat (for the more turbulent trip) at least once an hour.

317) USE THE HOTEL GYM!

If you are lucky enough to get a hotel with a gym USE IT! Hotels gyms are often a desert land that you can use as your play land! Get a workout in, even if it's not as much as you normally do. The weights and machines may be sparse or different than you are used to but not to worry, try some new exercises and change up the tempo. Change your tempo, hold different points of the movement, and be creative!

318) TIGHT SPACE EXERCISES!

Just because you don't have a lot of space in your room doesn't mean you can't take advantage of exercises that you know don't require much square footage! Sit-ups, push-ups, squats, planks, lunges, running in place, and jumping rope are all great for this. Jumping rope can be extremely efficient and won't take up much room in your luggage!

319) WATER, WATER, WATER!

Yes, I know I already mentioned this but you cannot underestimate the importance of water. When travelling we tend to forget about hydrating our bodies. Be sure to carry a water bottle with you wherever you go, you can easily get it refilled at café's, pubs, restaurants etc.

320) SWIM!

Swimming is an intense 'full body' workout; if you are staying somewhere with a pool or are close to a body of water, why not jump in for twenty minutes? It is guaranteed to tire you out and help you sleep better in the night!

321) PLAN YOUR DAYS!

It is useful to plan you day to know when your free time is! Try to fit in one mode of exercise EVERY DAY (even if it is just walking). Besides the health benefits of walking it will help save money that would otherwise be spent on public transport. If you are like most people and want to try all of the local food, I get it, I like food too; just try to walk to the places you like to mitigate some of the damage your food eating competition is going to do to your waistline.

322) USE YOUR PHONE!

Applications on your mobile phone really come into their own when you are in unfamiliar surroundings. Make the most of them to get around as well as using the apps that will help with your diet and exercise! You can get apps that tell you how far you have run and how quickly you ran it. This way you can still carry on trying to beat your personal best. How amazing does that sound?

323) HAVE FUN!

After all, this is your vacation so you have to go with the flow. There may be times where you don't eat a healthy dinner but you shouldn't feel guilty about it. Of course, if the healthy option is there then you should take it! Just remember the tips you have learned and embrace the experience!

So there it is; so far you have learnt A LOT of tips and hacks to help you on this new journey. For a finishing touch I have some miscellaneous tips and general health and life hacks that can help you on a day-to-day basis!

More Life Hacks

Ok so maybe the following life hacks won't necessarily 'save' your life, but they are great tips and tricks to improve your life.

324) WRIST WEIGHTS!

Like I have said before, there are ALWAYS opportunities to exercise, even little things you can do throughout the day to help. Try putting on wrist weights when completing simple tasks! When blow-drying your hair, decorating the house, or working in the yard! These everyday tasks can be put to good use if you add a wrist weights; you will soon feel and see the difference from this simple hack! Ankle weights work great too!

325) 20/20/20 RULE!

Eye strain is a huge problem nowadays, especially since we spend so much time in front of screens, but this rule should help to prevent any major problems. Doctors have suggested that you should take 20 seconds to look at something 20 feet away EVERY 20 minutes!

326) COLD SHOWERS!

Taking a cold shower helps to activate good fat (brown fat) to burn bad fat (white fat) as energy! Brown fat also helps to improve circulation as well as reduce inflammation and repairing muscles!

327) MOVE ABOUT WHEN YOU ARE AWAKE!

It is thought that we sit for over 9 HOURS a day! We then sleep for over 7 HOURS a day (ideally)! That leaves just EIGHT hours to do everything else so it vital that we make the most of this time and get the blood flowing to keep us healthy!

328) MEDITATE!

It is thought that 90% of ALL doctors' visits are due to stress; 90%! That is a HUGE amount, so we need to find a way to relax and meditation could be the key to this dilemma. Meditation can help you to slow down and allow you to reconnect with yourself on a personal level! Try downloading an app that teaches you how to meditate by simply following the directions.

329) SMELL AN ORANGE!
Everyone knows that an orange is a healthy option at any point during the day. However, just the smell of an orange is said to de-stress, improve your mood, and make you feel more awake in general!

330) RELAXING JOURNEY TO WORK!
Commuting to and from work is often seen as the most stressful part of the day, but it doesn't have to be this way! Try and use this time to relax, listen to your favorite music, audio book, or maybe even a meditation audio (just don't close your eyes while driving!). If we stress on our way home, we are less likely to complete any exercise when we get there because all we want to do is relax!

331) RELIEVE STRESS BY CLEANING!
Cleaning and organizing your home or car can be a great stress reliever as it makes you concentrate on something else! Why not stick on your favorite CD and dance the day away as you feel the stress draining from your body?

332) APPS, APPS, APPS!
The majority of the population now has smartphones and as a result, there are some fantastic apps being added regularly. Take advantage of this as they can be VERY helpful! There are apps that will help with your workouts, apps that will help you to count the calories, apps with delicious recipes; the list goes on and on!

333) WHITE TEETH!
There are so many options on the market when it comes to teeth whitening, many of which are fairly expensive. The best option may have been sitting right under your nose all this time and it's no monkey business! BANANA PEEL! Try rubbing the inside of a banana peel onto your teeth for about a minute each (top and bottom), leave for ten minutes and then brush off with a DRY toothbrush. If carried out regularly, you should see positive results soon enough!

334) TOOTHPASTE!

Toothpaste has found more uses than just teeth in the home in recent years, first it was discovered that putting toothpaste on a zit will help to remove it. Now, toothpaste is also being used to whiten fingernails! This could help if you are kicking the dirty habit of smoking; when mixed in with lemon juice (a natural bleaching agent), toothpaste can help to whiten yellow nails!

335) MOTIVATIONAL QUOTES!

There are thousands of motivational quotes in the world but it is time to use them to your advantage. Why not print some out and post them about the house or change your mobile phone background to one so you are constantly gaining inspiration. Your favorite song lyrics can also have the same effect! Here are a few of my favorites:

- "The trouble with not having a goal is that you can spend your life running up and down the field and never score." – *Bill Copeland*

- "It is never too late to be what you might have been." – *George Eliot*

- "All our dreams can come true – if we have the courage to pursue them." – *Walt Disney*

- "Great minds discuss ideas. Average minds discuss events. Small minds discuss people." – *Eleanor Roosevelt*

- "An eye for an eye only ends up making the whole world blind." – *M.K. Gandhi*

- "I haven't failed. I've just found 10,000 ways that won't work." – *Thomas Edison*

- "It is the mark of an educated mind to be able to entertain a thought without accepting it." – *Aristotle*

- "It's not whether you get knocked down, it's whether you get up." – *Vince Lombardi*

- "Logic will get you from A to B. Imagination will take you everywhere." – *Albert Einstein*

- "Never leave that till tomorrow which you can do today."
  - *Benjamin Franklin*

- "Even if you're on the right track, you'll get run over if you just sit there."
  - Will Rogers

336) GOOD POSTURE WHEN DRIVING!

Whether on a short journey or a long, one always tries to practice good posture when driving. This can help to prevent future health problems as it is very easy to cause a long-term back injury because of slouching when driving! Sit upright with your shoulders back, head forward, chest up, and keep your abs engaged with your belly button driven in towards your spine.

337) COMPLIMENTS ARE GOOD!

We all have something inside us which makes us vulnerable to compliments, but for some reason we aren't supposed to like or they make us feel uncomfortable; or worse accepting them could make us look conceded. WHY?? Compliments are a positive comment on the subject that the person has chosen to say something about. The next time someone says that you look good say thank you; I have been working my ass of in the gym, eating healthy, and taking care of myself! Own it and absorb it, and be proud of it!

338) KISS!

Many studies have looked at the impact of kissing when in a relationship and it is now thought to be more important than regular sex! People in less successful relationships experienced less kissing! So, if you have a partner, put this book down for a moment and go give them a kiss....tongue optional, but encouraged!

339) SLOW DOWN!

Many people get caught up in trying to do everything at once whether it's personal or work-related. Try to focus on one thing at a time and perfect that before you move on to something else. This can help to save time in the long run as you don't have to go back and fix previous mistakes!

340) COMMUNICATE!

Communication can be the key to a successful business AND personal life. Clear communication can help to make your work life more efficient as well as paving a more successful personal life; especially in relationship! Say what you mean and mean what you say!

341) TIME YOUR LIFE!

I bet that you would be surprised how much time you waste DAILY! For one day or maybe even one week, time your day and write down EVERYTHING you do. By doing this you can find parts of your day that are wasted. This can be a great way to make your days more efficient! I bet your excuse of 'I don't have time to work out,' or 'I don't have time to cook healthy' goes out the window when you find out how much time you have wasted (probably on your smartphones) in a day!

342) USE PUBLIC TOILETS!

Now, A LOT of people avoid public toilets but this can be detrimental to our health and will also contribute towards constipation! If you need the toilet and keep resisting the urge because you are not at home, you are more than likely going to get constipated! Now if you have been doing everything I told you in this book you should have stronger legs and core so you can always use the "hover" technique, just watch out for the splash! HA!

343) LOSE THE TV!

Ever heard the expression 'the more you watch, the less you know'? It didn't come around by chance; it actually means something and is completely true! People who watch more than two hours of TV a day are more likely to have a lower mental acuity score and are also more likely to be diagnosed with an attention disorder such as ADHD. This is because we are overloading the brain with rapid-fire stimuli! Your brain needs to slow down to learn how to process information in an orderly manner.

344) QUIT SMOKING EASILY!

If you have been attempting to stop smoking (which you should be if you aren't already) but are struggling, try visiting a sauna for the first few days! Besides it being a nice treat, you will sweat out the nicotine making it significantly easier to quit!

345) TUMS FOR ULCERS!

If you have a mouth ulcer that has been bothering you recently, try putting a tums on the ulcer, you should see and feel it disappear within HOURS!

346) ACNE PREVENTION!

Acne can be one of the most frustrating things around! I'm sure you have tried different creams and treatments out there, but a simple change our diet may be the answer. Any foods that are rich in omega-3 fatty acids will help to prevent acne. These include wild caught salmon, omega enriched eggs (yes the yolk), edamame, flax, beans, and walnuts!

347) CHEW GUM IN AN EXAM!

The day has finally come for your big exam and you are worried that you won't remember all that you have learned. Try chewing on the SAME FLAVOR gum that you chewed on when studying; this is meant to send triggers to our brain and help us to recall what we have learned!

348) DIY HAIR REMOVAL!

Wouldn't it be nice to not have to worry about constantly removing unwanted hair? Now you can! All you need is some coffee grounds and some baking soda. Mix in 2 tablespoons of coffee grounds with one teaspoon of baking soda and dab onto the area of which you wish to remove hair. Try doing this for a few days, the baking soda intensifies the compounds of the coffee which breaks down the hair follicles right down to the root!

349) WATER TO REMEMBER DREAMS!

I bet you have spent a few moments on the edge of the bed one morning trying to remember your dreams from the night before! We have ALL done it at some point.

Now we may have a way to remember them more frequently. Try drinking half a glass of water before you go to bed and then repeat this as you wake up, this will act as a psychological cue to remember our dreams!

350) WHITER TEETH!

So the first trick was to use the banana peel on your teeth but there is a second tip that I would like to share with you. For this, you will need strawberries and baking soda (all will be explained). First, mash up one or two strawberries, add half a teaspoon of baking soda and mix together until you have a paste. Then, apply the paste to your teeth using your finger or a toothbrush; leave it on for around 4-5 minutes and rinse. After a few applications, you should really start to see a difference; however, it isn't recommended that you do this too often as the baking soda can erode enamel!

351) ANNOYING ITCHY THROAT?

An itchy throat can be so frustrated because your tongue only reaches the tip of the itch and you can be left feeling uncomfortable and irritated. A good tip for this is to scratch your ear. By doing this you are stimulating your ear, creating a reflection in your throat which causes a slight muscle spasm and completely KILLS that annoying itch!

352) MAKE YOUR LEGS CAMERA READY!

Make your legs look great in a picture...STOP leg training a week or two before! If you have a photo shoot coming up or want to look great in your swimsuit...or birthday suit? Stop doing resistance leg training like squats, lunges, and more a week beforehand. This is practice bodybuilders and physique competitors do, including myself, when I have a shoot. Giving your legs a week off of training allows the muscles to come through as they aren't full of so much blood and glycogen.

353) WATER TAPERING!

Do you have a vacation or photo shoot coming up where you want to look a little leaner? Try drinking a LOT of water a week or two out from the day where you will be showing your goods. This is a trick I use before photoshoots and bodybuilders use before going on stage. A week or two out start drinking more water than you are used to, let's say about 1 gallon. Each day after that slowly taper your water down until the day before you are only drinking about half of a gallon of water. What does this do? It takes your body a couple of days to reach equilibrium, so by drinking lots of water you will be excreting more water than you are taking in. Eventually when you get down to the last day your water intake will be lower, but your body will be excreting water at higher rate through urine and fecal matter. As a result, our skin will be tighter with less fluid covering your abs and the scale will be down a few pounds. *Now remember the scale will be down but it will most likely be due to a loss of water, probably not much fat, but what the hell, you look great! This is NOT meant to make you dehydrated, this is simply meant to make your body excrete excess water and get used to drinking more high quality H2O!

354) PINTEREST!

Pinterest is an extremely helpful app that will allow you to find great workout tips and healthy recipes; if you find one that you like, you can 'pin' it to your board and save it for later!

355) SWEAR!

F**K!!! Research has actually shown that people who swear when in pain have a higher pain tolerance (plus it can feel good to get it out of your system, right?). Less perceived pain will lead to a lower heart rate! So next time you stub your toe on that bookshelf that you walk into daily (because you forget it there), don't be afraid to shout a little (or big) swear word! Be careful where you use this tip though, it may be best to be left just for the home (sh**!) [2].

356) FIX A BLISTER!

Blisters can be the bane of your life if you get them regularly but here is a trick to lessen the pain. As soon as you start to feel the early signs of a blister, apply some duct tape (try to avoid any creases). This will soften the area and reduce pain; many runners swear by it and find it better than simply applying a bandage as it stays on better!

357) TIGHTEN SKIN WITH EPSOM SALT BATH!

Bathe your way to tight skin! Another crazy trick celebrity, bodybuilders, and even my crazy ass self has done is to take a baking soda bath! Bathe in 2 cups of Epsom salt (or a couple boxes of baking soda) in hot water for about 30 minutes and your skin will be tight! Epsom salt or baking soda is a safe and inexpensive way to neutralize your body and detoxify from the typical western diet of fried foods and high acid consumption, alcohol, caffeine, nicotine, and medications.

358) HEMORRHOID CREAM AND SARAN WRAP FOR YOUR ABS!

LOL, this actually works! Want your abs to show but have a little water covering them? Get them showing with some hemorrhoid cream and saran wrap! – What?!! If you want to lose water from your skin to look great the next day, get a bottle of hemorrhoid cream. Hemorrhoid cream is used to pull fluid out of hemorrhoids and it works in the same manner on your abs! Slather your stomach and back with it (may be best to test a small area beforehand for any allergic reaction), then saran wrap around your torso and go to bed. Now this isn't the most restful sleep you will ever have, but you will wake up with a pool of sweat collected in the wrap and your skin will be tighter (at least for the day!) Side note: if you like sweating, rub some hemorrhoid cream on your stomach and back before you go for a run or workout in the gym and you will be sweating up a storm in no time. *Btw if you have a lot of fat covering your abs this will not work; you need to be pretty lean to see a significant difference, although if you simply want to sweat a little go for it!

359) HACK YOUR ICE TRAY!

Ice trays can be used for other things besides ice….wow! Try blending up some fresh fruit that is about to go bad, place in the ice tray and freeze. This way you can add the fruit ice to your water for flavor or add to your greens smoothies for some sweetness. Another great option is to freeze lemon or lime juice and use the lemon/lime ice cubes to freshen up your tea or beverage of choice.

360) MIRACLE FRUIT!

Have you ever wanted to eat something sweet but didn't want the calories or guilt…. of course you have! Well now there is a solution that actually makes sour foods taste sweet and it's called the miracle fruit! This fruit is grown from an evergreen shrub in West Africa and has a myriad of names: like Fruit Miracle, Miracle Berry, and Sweet Berry to name a few. How does it work? The fruit contains a chemical that affects the taste receptors in the tongue and cause anything sour to taste sweet! Simply eat some of this fruit before you want your sweet fix and then bite into something that is slightly sour or bitter (like grapefruit, lemon, balsamic vinegar, pickles, bell peppers, carrots, goat cheese, etc.) and taste the sweet joy of this little miracle fruit!

361) ACHY FEET? USE A BALL!

Have you ever had it where the bottoms of your feet start to hurt? This is because the fibrous tissue running from your heel to your toes called the fascia gets really tight. Essentially this needs to be massaged out and if you don't have a massage therapist around, grab a golf ball or tennis ball and roll it from your heel to your toes for a few minutes. This will stretch out and massage the fascia and alleviate the tension. You can also freeze a water bottle and use this the same way to get some cold relief at the same time, bonus!

362) SNEEZE PLEASE!

Have you ever been in a public place and tried to hold back that sneeze or yawn to be 'polite'? We all have, but doing this can cause the fluids that need to escape our noses, hence having to cover our mouths, get thrown back into our sinuses. Similarly, if you hold back a yawn you limit your brain from being cooled when it's overheated. So next time someone looks at you for yawning or sneezing too loud, let them know your health depends on it!

363) HATE CROWDS, AVOID THEM AT OFF PEAK TIMES!

Gyms can be an intimidating place so why not help yourself out and go when it's not as busy? Go to the gym when there's less of a chance for people to be there like early in the morning, late morning, early afternoon (after the lunch crowd), and later at night. Get yourself acclimated to the gym, the equipment, and the people then you can slowly work your way through the after work crowds with confidence!

364) CAFFEINE FREE WEEKEND!

What, what, what?! I know, I know, I love my coffee and caffeine as much as anyone but you eventually need more and more to get your caffeine fix! Try taking the weekend off from caffeine to bring your tolerance down a touch and you can look forward to your morning cup of Joe…..while reading this book by Joe-y!

365) LOVE!

This is the last hack for a reason. You need to allow LOVE in your life, let those around you LOVE you; allow people to care for you, worry about you, simply be there for you! Allow yourself to LOVE others as giving love is just as important as getting love. Lastly, LOVE yourself! You just read this entire book (hopefully) and you need to be proud of yourself that you have taken the time to become a healthier and better you!

BONUS: 'RIPPED' RECIPES

*Nutritional values (per serving) are estimates only and will vary.

MEDITERRANEAN QUINOA SALAD

INGREDIENTS:

- ✓ 1 cup dry quinoa
- ✓ ¼ cup crumbled feta cheese
- ✓ 10 Kalamata olives, halved
- ✓ 1 tbsp. fresh basil, chopped
- ✓ 2 cups spinach, chopped
- ✓ 1 tbsp. fresh parsley, chopped
- ✓ 1 cup chopped asparagus
- ✓ 1 tbsp. fresh oregano, chopped

- ✓ 1 cup garbanzo beans (chick peas)
- ✓ 5 tbsp. extra virgin olive oil
- ✓ 1 cup grape tomatoes, halved
- ✓ 5 tbsp. red wine vinegar
- ✓ ½ cup red pepper, chopped
- ✓ 1 tbsp. Dijon mustard
- ✓ ¼ cup red onion, chopped
- ✓ Sea salt and ground pepper to taste

INSTRUCTIONS: 1. In a saucepan, combine quinoa and 2 cups water. Bring to a boil. Reduce heat, cover, and simmer until liquid evaporates — about 15-20 min. Remove from heat, allow cooling, and placing in a large bowl. 2. Whisk together extra virgin olive oil, red wine vinegar, Dijon mustard, salt, & pepper and set aside. 3. Once quinoa is cool, add remaining ingredients and gently toss. Serves 4.

NUTRITIONAL VALUE: Calories: 480, Protein: 13g, Carbs: 55g, Fat: 25g

SOUTHWESTERN QUINOA SALAD

INGREDIENTS:

- ✓ 1 cup uncooked quinoa,
- ✓ 1 15oz. can low-sodium black beans
- ✓ 1 cup grape tomatoes, halved
- ✓ 1 red bell pepper chopped
- ✓ ¼ cup finely chopped red onion
- ✓ 1 jalapeno pepper, finely chopped
- ✓ ¼ cup chopped fresh cilantro
- ✓ Juice of 1 large (or 2 small) limes
- ✓ 2 tbsp. extra virgin olive oil
- ✓ season with sea salt and pepper

INSTRUCTIONS: 1. Place quinoa in a saucepan with 2 cups water. Bring to a boil, then cover and simmer for 10-15 minutes, until the water is absorbed. 2. Place cooled cooked quinoa in a salad bowl with the black beans, tomatoes, red onion, peppers, and cilantro. 3. Whisk lime juice, oil, salt & pepper in a small bowl & drizzle over salad. Makes 4 servings.

NUTRITIONAL VALUE: Calories: 318, Protein: 12.25g, Carbs: 50g, Fat: 7g

CHICKEN AND BROWN RICE

INGREDIENTS:

- ✓ 1 cup uncooked brown rice
- ✓ 2 grilled chicken breasts, sliced
- ✓ ¼ cup water
- ✓ 1 tablespoon low sodium taco seasoning
- ✓ 1 sliced red pepper
- ✓ ¼ cup sliced avocado
- ✓ ½ diced onion
- ✓ 1 cup black beans
- ✓ ½ cup salsa

INSTRUCTIONS: 1. Cook rice according to instructions. 2. Add water to a skillet and bring to a boil. Add diced vegetables and taco seasoning and simmer for 5 min. 3. Add chicken, black beans and rice. 4. Add salsa and heat for another 1-2 min. 5. Top with shredded cheese and a slice of avocado before serving. Makes 4 servings.

NUTRITIONAL VALUE: Calories: 350, Protein: 50g, Carb: 34g, Fat: 3.5g

MEDITERRANEAN CHICKEN

INGREDIENTS:

- ✓ 2 teaspoons olive oil
- ✓ 2 tablespoons white wine
- ✓ 3 cloves garlic, minced
- ✓ 6 skinless, boneless chicken breast halves
- ✓ ½ cup diced onion
- ✓ 3 cups tomatoes, chopped
- ✓ ½ cup white wine
- ✓ 2 teaspoons chopped fresh thyme
- ✓ 1 tablespoon chopped fresh basil
- ✓ ½ cup Kalamata olives
- ✓ ¼ cup chopped fresh parsley
- ✓ salt and pepper to taste

INSTRUCTIONS: 1. Heat the oil and 2 tbsp. white wine in a large skillet (med heat). Add chicken and sauté about 4 to 6 min each side, until golden. Remove chicken from skillet and set aside. 2. Sauté garlic in pan drippings for 30 seconds, then add onion and sauté for 3 min. Add tomatoes and bring to a boil. Lower heat, add ½ cup white wine and simmer for 10 min. Add thyme and basil and simmer for 5 more min. 3. Return chicken to skillet and cover. Cook over low heat until the chicken is cooked through and no longer pink inside. 4. Add olives and parsley to the skillet and cook for 1 min. Season with salt and pepper to taste and serve.

NUTRITIONAL VALUE: Calories: 222, Protein: 28g, Carbs: 7g, Fat: 6g

QUINOA CHICKEN

INGREDIENTS:

- ✓ 24oz. of cooked chicken breast
- ✓ 2 cups of uncooked quinoa
- ✓ 1 cup chopped raw onion
- ✓ Jalapeno to taste (optional)

INSTRUCTIONS: 1. Boil 4 cups of water in a bowl, once at a boil add the quinoa and bring to a medium heat, cook until a little water is remaining in the quinoa. Turn off the heat and cover the quinoa for 10 minutes. 2. Add remaining ingredients in with the quinoa after 10 minutes, season to taste and divide into 5 portions. Serves 5 people. (Recipe also great with Shrimp)

NUTRITIONAL VALUE: Calories: 435, Protein: 40g, Carbs: 50g, Fat: 6g

SALMON BURGERS

INGREDIENTS:

- ✓ 1 whole egg
- ✓ 1 salmon fillet, shredded
- ✓ 2 egg whites
- ✓ 1/3 cup raw oatmeal
- ✓ 1 teaspoon minced garlic
- ✓ 2 tablespoons freshly chopped parsley
- ✓ 1 tablespoon olive oil

INSTRUCTIONS: 1. In a bowl, combine salmon, eggs, oatmeal, parsley, and garlic until well blended. Form mixture into patties about 1/2 inches thick. 2. Heat oil in a skillet on medium heat & place each patty on the pan. Cook patties for 4 min, flip, and then cook for another 2-3 min. 3. Serve with a wholegrain bun or lettuce wrap.

NUTRITIONAL VALUE: Calories: 512, Protein: 33.4g, Carb: 35.8g, Fat: 26.4g

THAI SPICY CHICKEN

INGREDIENTS:

- ✓ 6 chicken breasts cut in half
- ✓ 12oz natural non-fat or low-fat yogurt
- ✓ 2-3 tbsp. Thai red curry paste
- ✓ 4 tbsp. chopped fresh cilantro
- ✓ About a 3 inch piece cucumber

INSTRUCTIONS: 1.Preheat your oven to 375°f (350°f fan oven). Place the chicken into a shallow dish in one layer. Blend one third of the yogurt, all of the curry paste, and only three tbsp. of the cilantro. Season the mixture with salt and coat the chicken evenly on both sides. Let the chicken marinate for a minimum of 10 minutes or leave in the refrigerator overnight. 2. Cook the chicken for 35-40 minutes until they are a golden brown color. 3. For a dipping sauce blend the excess yogurt and cilantro together & add chopped cucumber. Serves 4-5.

NUTRITIONAL VALUE: Calories: 266, Protein: 43g, Carbs: 8g, Fat: 3g

CILANTRO LIME FISH TACOS

INGREDIENTS:

- ✓ 1 lb. white fish (wild caught), rinsed and pat dried
- ✓ 1 tsp olive oil
- ✓ 1 small onion, chopped
- ✓ 4 garlic cloves, finely minced
- ✓ 2 jalapeño peppers, chopped
- ✓ 2 cups diced tomatoes
- ✓ 1/4 cup fresh cilantro, chopped
- ✓ 3 tbsp. lime juice
- ✓ 8 5-inch white corn tortillas
- ✓ 1 medium avocado, sliced
- ✓ salt and pepper to taste

INSTRUCTIONS: 1. Heat olive oil in a skillet. Sauté onion until translucent & add garlic. 2. Place fish on the skillet and cook until fish flakes. 3. Add jalapeño peppers, tomatoes, cilantro and lime juice. Sauté over medium-high heat for about 5 minutes, breaking up the fish with the spoon to get everything mixed well; season to taste with salt and pepper. 4. Serve a little over 1/4 cup of fish on each warmed tortillas with a slice or 2 of avocado and enjoy!

NUTRITIONAL VALUE (2 tacos): Calories: 319, Protein: 26.5g, Carbs: 33.7g, Fat: 12g

HERB MUSTARD GLAZED SALMON

INGREDIENTS:

- ✓ 2 garlic cloves
- ✓ 1/4 tsp finely chopped rosemary leaves
- ✓ 3/4 tsp finely chopped thyme leaves
- ✓ 1 tbsp. dry white wine
- ✓ 1 tbsp. extra-virgin olive oil
- ✓ 2 tbsp. Dijon mustard
- ✓ 2 tbsps. wholegrain mustard
- ✓ Nonstick olive oil cooking spray
- ✓ 6 (6 to 8-ounce) salmon fillets
- ✓ 6 lemon wedges

INSTRUCTIONS: 1. In a mini food processor, combine garlic, rosemary, thyme, wine, oil, Dijon mustard, & whole-grain mustard. Grind the mustard sauce until combined. 2. Line a heavy rimmed baking sheet with foil & nonstick spray. 3. Arrange the salmon fillets on the baking sheet and sprinkle them with salt and pepper. Broil for 2 minutes. Spoon the mustard sauce over the fillets. Continue broiling until the fillets are just cooked through& golden brown, about 5 min longer. Serves 6.

NUTRITION VALUE: Calories: 294, Protein: 45g, Carbs: 3g, Fat: 11g

CHEESY VEGGIE MEDLEY SCRAMBLER

INGREDIENTS:

- ✓ 5 large egg whites
- ✓ ½ of white onion, finely chopped
- ✓ 2 whole eggs
- ✓ 4 tablespoons cottage cheese
- ✓ 1 cup diced cucumbers
- ✓ Shredded low fat mozzarella cheese
- ✓ ½ cup chopped mushroom
- ✓ Season with cracked black pepper

INSTRUCTIONS: 1. Place the eggs and egg whites in a bowl and whisk together. In a frying pan, cook the mushrooms and onions until they are soft. Remove from frying pan. 2. Add the egg mixture with all of the ingredients (add the shredded cheese now or sprinkle on later) into the frying pan with a tablespoon of olive oil or avocado oil and cook to your liking.

*If you would like extra carbs feel free to add some whole grain toast, brown rice, or quinoa.

NUTRITIONAL VALUE: Calories: 375, Protein: 45g, Carbs: 20g, Fat: 19g

MEDITERRANEAN SCRAMBLER

INGREDIENTS:

- ✓ 3 whole eggs
- ✓ 1 cup chopped tomatoes
- ✓ 2 cups fresh spinach
- ✓ 2 large fresh basil leaves
- ✓ Goat cheese (sprinkle on top)
- ✓ Cracked black pepper

INSTRUCTIONS: 1. Scramble eggs to liking, add tomatoes and spinach. 2. Remove from pan, sprinkle goat cheese and chopped basil on top.

NUTRIONAL VALUE: Calories: 337, Protein: 27g, Carbs: 11g, Fat: 21g

GROUND TURKEY SCRAMBLER

INGREDIENTS:

- ✓ 4oz 93% lean ground turkey
- ✓ 1 cup spinach
- ✓ 4 whole eggs
- ✓ Feta cheese

INSTRUCTIONS: 1. Cook the ground turkey in a separate pan. 2. In a bowl whisk the eggs and place in a medium heat frying pan coated with olive oil or avocado oil. 3. Mix in spinach and ground turkey in with cooked eggs. 4. Sprinkle on feta cheese.

NUTRITIONAL VALUE: Calories: 477, Protein: 50g, Carbs: 2g, Fat: 28g

SALMON SALAD

INGREDIENTS:

- ✓ 1 salmon filet
- ✓ 1/3 cup Greek yogurt
- ✓ ½ teaspoon minced garlic
- ✓ ½ teaspoon fresh dill
- ✓ ¼ cup finely diced onions

INSTRUCTIONS: 1. In a bowl, mix together Greek yogurt, minced garlic, dill, and diced onions. 2. Add salmon and stir until salad is formed. Makes 2 servings.

NUTRITIONAL VALUE: Calories: 89, Protein: 22.5g, Carbs: 3g, Fat: 8g

POWER PROTEIN BARS AND SHAKES

NO BAKE ALMOND PROTEIN BARS

INGREDIENTS:

- ✓ 4 servings Whey Protein Powder
- ✓ 1/2 cup Organic Nut Butter
- ✓ 3/4 cup slivered or whole almonds
- ✓ 3/4 cup Milk (or milk substitute)
- ✓ 3 cups Oats

INSTRUCTIONS: Combine all ingredients in a bowl and mix well. Spread in a 9x9 baking pan lined with parchment paper. Place in the refrigerator and allow to set overnight. Cut into 6 equal squares.*You may also use chocolate whey protein powder instead of strawberry. Makes 6 protein bars.

NUTRITIONAL VALUE: Calories: 539, Protein: 35g, Carbs: 47g, Fat: 25g

CHOCOLATE ALMOND BUTTER PROTEIN BARS

INGREDIENTS:

- ✓ 2 servings Chocolate Whey Protein Powder,
- ✓ 3 Bananas, Medium
- ✓ 3 tbsp. Creamy Almond butter
- ✓ 1 ounce Honey
- ✓ 2 cups Oats
- ✓ 4 ounces Skim Milk
- ✓ 5 Egg Whites
- ✓ 1.5 tsp Cinnamon

INSTRUCTIONS: 1. Preheat your oven to 350 degrees F. 2. Place the oats in a blender until they reach a flour-like texture. 3. Place the oats in a mixing bowl and add in the cinnamon and protein powder. Next add in the peanut butter and mix thoroughly. Mash your bananas and add them to this mixture, along with the honey and egg whites. Mix well. Finally, add the skim milk and mix again. 4. Pour batter into a 9x9 or 9x13 greased baking pan. Bake for 15 to 20 minutes, or until a toothpick comes out clean from the center of the pan. Allow the bars to cool and then cut into 6 bars.

NUTRITIONAL VALUE: Calories: 375, Protein: 25g, Carbs: 40g, Fat: 8g

CHOCOLATE BANANA WALNUT PROTEIN BARS

INGREDIENTS:

- ✓ 1.5 Cups Instant Oatmeal
- ✓ 3 Medium Bananas, Mashed
- ✓ 5 Servings of Chocolate Protein Powder (or flavor of choice)
- ✓ 4 Egg Whites
- ✓ 1/2 Cup Walnuts, Ground
- ✓ 1 tablespoon Vanilla Extract
- ✓ 1 tablespoon Cinnamon

INSTRUCTIONS: 1. In a large bowl, add all dry ingredients (oats, protein, walnuts, cinnamon) mix all ingredients in a bowl/stir. 2. Scoop mixture into a 9x9 Pyrex dish and bake at 350 degrees F for 15 minutes. Makes 8-9 Bars.

NUTRITIONAL VALUE: Calories: 204, Protein: 16g, Carbs: 22g, Fat: 7g

ALMOND BANANA PROTEIN SHAKE

INGREDIENTS:

- ✓ 1 medium banana
- ✓ 1 cup plain yogurt
- ✓ 8 oz. ice cold water
- ✓ 1 ounce ground almonds
- ✓ 1 cup raw oats
- ✓ 1 serving protein powder (flavor of choice)

INSTRUCTIONS: Place all ingredients in a blender and enjoy.

NUTRITIONAL VALUE: Calories: 650, Protein: 50g, Carbs: 75g, Fat: 17g

BERRY PROTEIN SHAKE

INGREDIENTS:

- ✓ 8oz. water
- ✓ 1 cup blueberries (substitute any berries)
- ✓ 1 serving protein powder (flavor of choice)

INSTRUCTIONS: Blend to desired consistency.

NUTRITIONAL VALUE: Calories: 350, Protein: 46g, Carbs: 25g, Fat: 3g

CINNAMON BANANA OAT PROTEIN SHAKE

INGREDIENTS:

- ✓ 8oz. milk or milk alternative
- ✓ 1 medium banana
- ✓ 1/2 cup raw oats
- ✓ 1 serving of whey protein (may vary with brand)
- ✓ cinnamon to flavor

INSTRUCTIONS: Place all ingredients in a blender and enjoy. *Tip: Substitute water for milk to decrease caloric intake

NUTRITIONAL VALUE: Calories: 554, Protein: 60g, Carbs: 68g, Fat: 6g

COCONUT WATER PROTEIN SHAKE

INGREDIENTS:

- ✓ 12oz. pure coconut water
- ✓ 1 serving protein powder, (flavor of choice)

INSTRUCTIONS: Place in shaker container, shake, and enjoy.

NUTRITIONAL VALUE: Calories: 320g, Protein: 47g, Carbs: 21g, Fat: 5g

DRINK YOUR GREENS PEANUT BUTTER PROTEIN SHAKE

INGREDIENTS:

- ✓ 8-16oz. water
- ✓ 1 serving protein powder
- ✓ 1 cup fresh spinach (or other greens)
- ✓ 2 tablespoons all natural peanut butter (may add any other nut butter you please)

INSTRUCTIONS: Combine ingredients and blend away!

NUTRITIONAL VALUE: Calories: 460, Protein: 53g, Carbs: 12g, Fat: 23g

So there you have it! ALL the tips you could possibly ever want and need to make this change a positive one and to become the person you WANT to be. Be sure to keep this book as a reference to check back on. Remember to stay STRONG and POSITIVE. Work hard and you WILL become the person you want to be. You WILL achieve your goals! GOOD LUCK!!!

If you want a complete nutrition and/or complete workout plan you can find a Renovation Plan on my site www.TheLifestyleRenovation.com

TO YOUR LIFE,
Joey Thurman
@JoeyThurmanFit

REFERENCES

[1]http://journals.lww.com/nsca-scj/Abstract/2012/10000/
Exercise_as_a_Management_Strategy_for_the.7.aspx

[2] - http://journals.lww.com/neuroreport/Pages/default.aspx?PAPNotFound=true

[3] - http://www.pponline.co.uk/encyc/
sport-psychology-encouragement-boosts-performance-113#

[4] - http://www.ncbi.nlm.nih.gov/pubmed/24954193

[5] - http://www.fasebj.org/cgi/content/meeting_abstract/20/4/A618-c

[6] - http://www.ncbi.nlm.nih.gov/pubmed/21669584

[7] - http://www.sciencedaily.com/releases/2010/09/100907104248.htm

[8] - http://www.ncbi.nlm.nih.gov/pmc/articles/PMC3119836/

[9]https://sleepfoundation.org/sites/default/files/sleepinamericapoll/SIAP_2011_
Summary_of_Findings.pdf

[10] -http://www.sleepforscience.org/stuff/contentmgr/files/8ed8b627e1f-
3848d6160a9c2a87f13b5/pdf/carskadon_dement_1980.pdf

[11] http://www.ncbi.nlm.nih.gov/pubmed/23832433

[12] http://www.ncbi.nlm.nih.gov/pubmed/23832433

[13] http://www.ncbi.nlm.nih.gov/pmc/articles/PMC3195546/

[14] http://www.webmd.com/vitamins-supple-
ments/ingredientmono-1073-WHEATGRASS.
aspx?activeIngredientId=1073&activeIngredientName=WHEATGRASS

[15] http://news.cancerconnect.com/whats-so-super-about-supergreens/

[16] http://articles.mercola.com/sites/articles/archive/2011/07/01/spirulina-the-amazing-super-food-youve-never-heard-of.aspx

[17] http://www.cdc.gov/HeartDisease/facts.htm

[18] http://time.com/3602415/sleep-problems-room-temperature/

[19] http://www.ncbi.nlm.nih.gov/pubmed/17332159

[20] http://www.ncbi.nlm.nih.gov/pubmed/23013520

[21] Chan, H., Burns, S. Oxygen consumption, substrate oxidation, and blood pressure following sprint interval exercise. Applied Physiology, Nutrition, and Metabolism. 2013. 38(2), 182-187.

[22] Heydari, M., et al. The effect of high-intensity intermittent exercise on body composition of overweight young males. Journal of Obesity. 2012. 480467. doi: 10.1155/2012/480467.

[23] Esbjornsson, M., et al. Greater growth hormone and insulin response in women than in men during repeated bouts of sprint exercise. Acta Physiology. 2009. 197(2), 107-115.[24] Schuenke, M., Mikat, R., et al. Effect of an Acute Period of Resistance Exercise on EPOC Implications for Body Mass Management. 2002. 86, 411-417.[25] http://www.jnutbio.com/article/S0955-2863%2814%2900208-3/abstract

[26] http://www.ncbi.nlm.nih.gov/pubmed/15724698

[27] http://www.eurekalert.org/pub_releases/2011-04/imc-sfr033111.php

[28] http://conditioningresearch.blogspot.com/2012/10/fasted-training-exercise-with-low.html

[29] Bowe WP & Logan AC. Acne vulgaris, probiotics and the gut-brain-skin axis – back to the future? Gut Pathogens 2011;3:1.

[30] http://www.ncbi.nlm.nih.gov/pubmed/11507179

[31] http://www.ncbi.nlm.nih.gov/pubmed/23919405

[32] http://www.ncbi.nlm.nih.gov/pubmed/23929734

[33] http://www.ncbi.nlm.nih.gov/pubmed/10722779

[34] http://www.prevention.com/weight-loss/food-chemicals-and-weight-gain

[35] http://www.prevention.com/food/dirtiest-produce-highest-levels-pesticides

[36] http://nutritionj.biomedcentral.com/articles/10.1186/1475-2891-3-9

[37] http://press.endocrine.org/doi/abs/10.1210/jc.2003-031855

[38] http://www.jstor.org/stable/20182250?seq=1#page_scan_tab_contents

[39] http://www.ncbi.nlm.nih.gov/pmc/articles/PMC3279464/

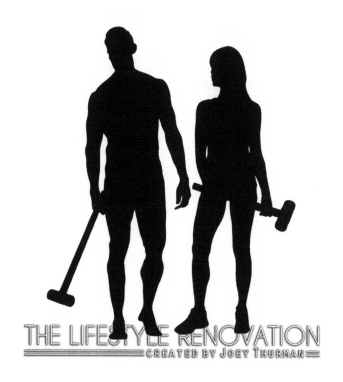

THELIFESTYLERENOVATION.COM